D1827586

My Diabetic Pressure Pot Recipe Book

Don't Miss These Healthy and Easy Recipes to Make Incredible Your Diabetic Diet

Cassandra Lane

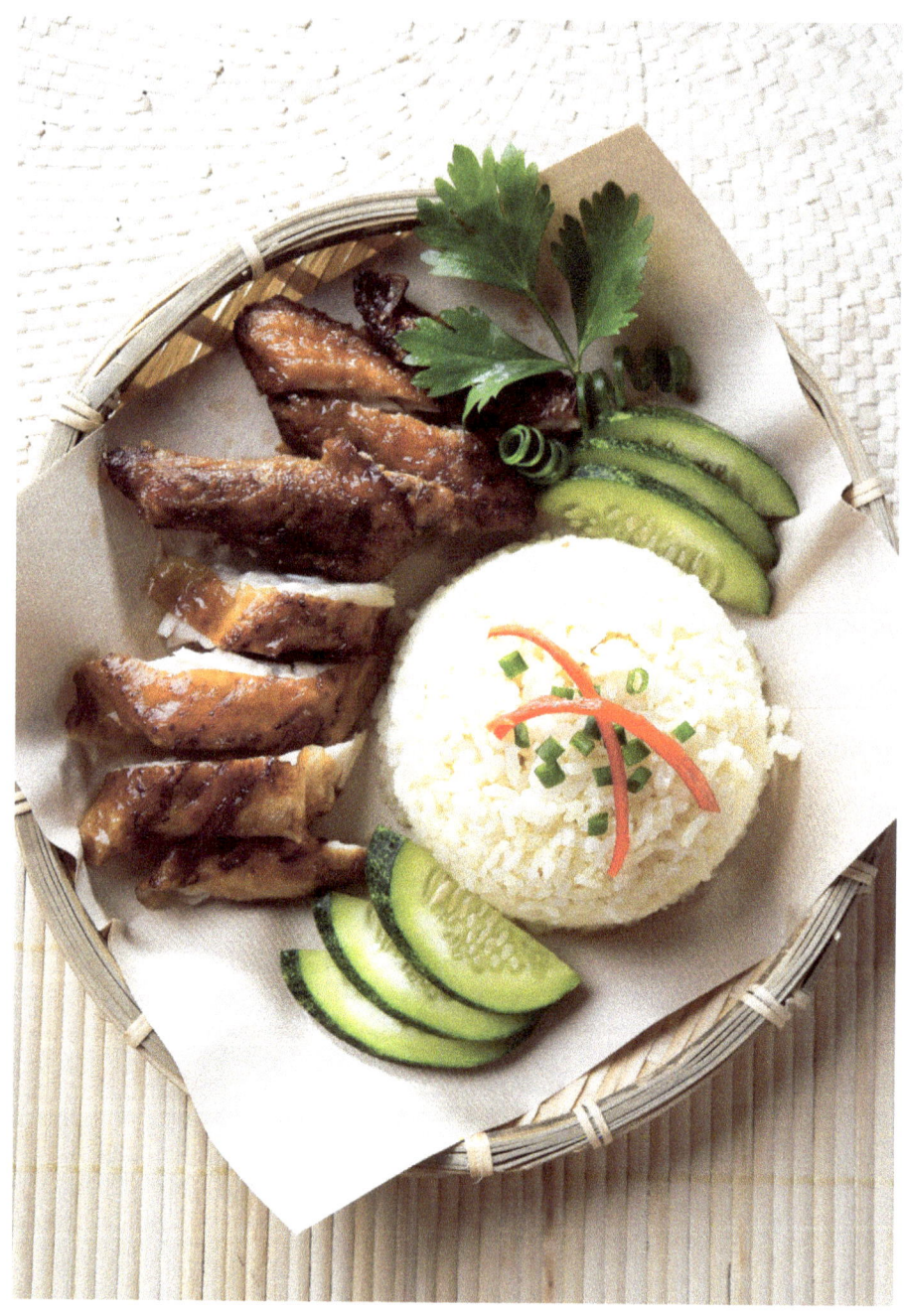

direct or indirect, which are incurred as a result of the use of information contained within this document, including, but not limited to, — errors, omissions, or inaccuracies.

Table of Contents

Chicken Liver Curry

Servings: 2

Cooking Time: 35 Minutes

Ingredients:

- 1lb diced chicken breast
- 0.5lb diced chicken liver
- 1lb chopped vegetables
- 1 cup broth
- 3tbsp curry paste

Directions:

1. Mix all the ingredients in your Pressure Pot.

2. Cook on Stew for 35 minutes.

3. Release the pressure naturally.

4. Nutrition Info: Per serving: Calories: 350; Carbs: 10; Sugar: 2 ; Fat: 17 ; Protein: 52 ; GL: 4

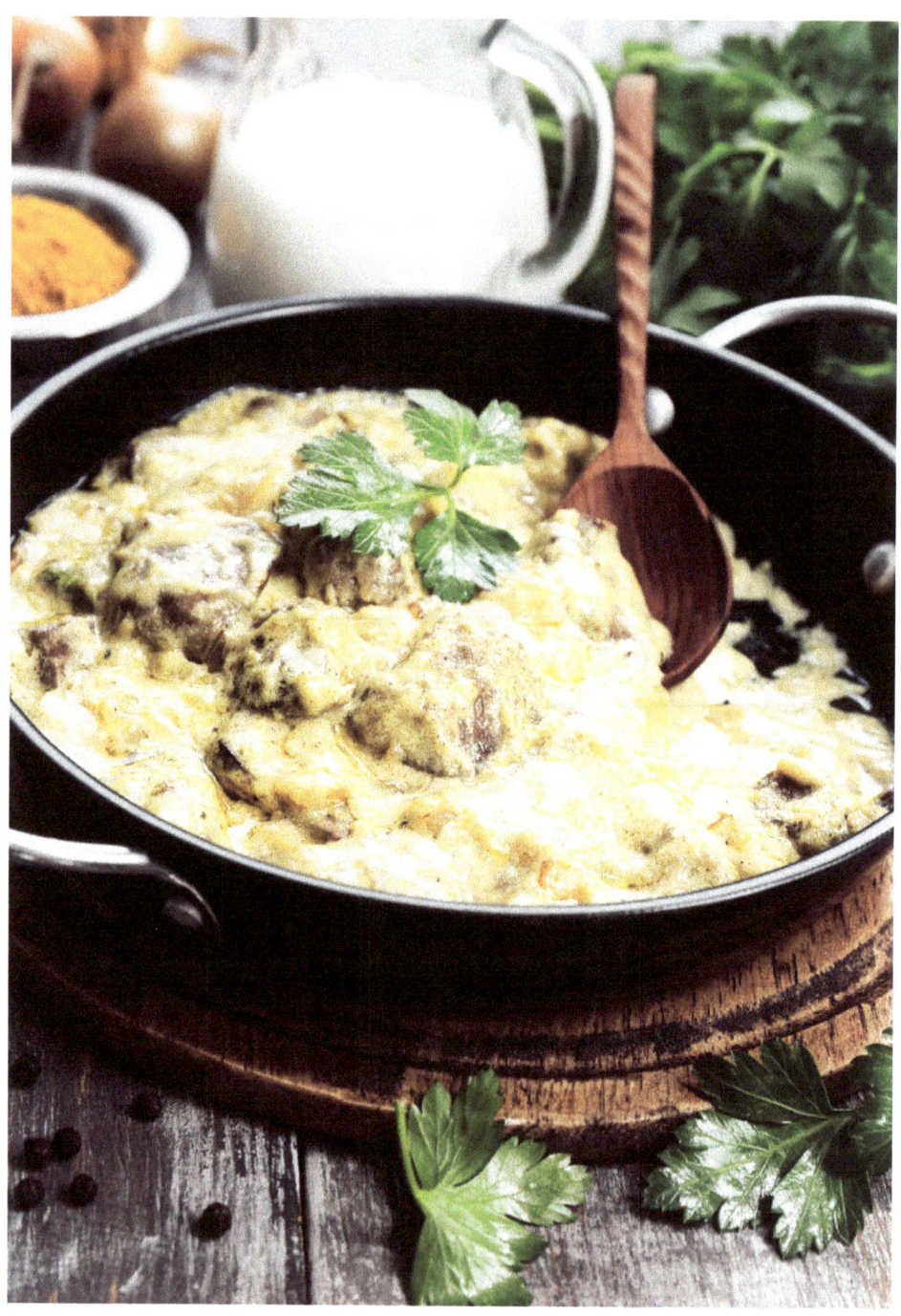

Spaghetti and Turkey Meatballs

Servings: 6

Cooking Time: 10 Minutes

Ingredients:

• 1 recipe (about 22) frozen Italian Turkey Sausage Meatballs

• 8 ounces whole grain thin spaghetti (uncooked), broken in half

• 1 tablespoon extra-virgin olive oil

• 1 (24-ounce) jar pasta sauce or 3 cups homemade sauce

• Freshly grated Parmesan cheese, for serving (optional)

Directions:

1. In the electric pressure cooker, arrange the frozen meatballs in a single layer. (Depending on the size of your meatballs and the size of your EPC, you may need more or less than 22.)

2. Place the broken spaghetti on top of the meatballs in an even layer. Drizzle the olive oil all over the spaghetti.

3. Pour in cups of water and the pasta sauce. If the

spaghetti is not completely covered, add a
bit more water. Do not stir.

4. Close and lock the lid of the pressure cooker. Set the valve to sealing.

5. Cook on high pressure for 10 minutes.

6. When the cooking is complete, hit Cancel and quick release the pressure.

7. Once the pin drops, unlock and remove the lid.

8. Serve with Parmesan cheese (if using).

9. Nutrition Info: Per serving: Calories: 47 Total Fat: 21g; Protein: 31g; Carbohydrates: 45g; Sugars: 8g; Fiber: 7g; Sodium: 1237mg

Sweet & Sour Brussels Sprout

Servings: 6

Cooking Time: 4 Minutes

Ingredients:

• 2 pounds Brussels sprouts, trimmed

• 2 tablespoons yacon syrup

• 3 tablespoons fresh lemon juice

• 2 tablespoons olive oil

• Salt and ground black pepper, as required

Directions:

1. In the pot of Pressure Pot, place all ingredients and stir to combine.

2. Close the lid and place the pressure valve to "Seal" position.

3. Press "Manual" and cook under "High Pressure" for about 4 minutes.

4. Press "Cancel" and carefully allow a "Quick" release.

5. Open the lid and stir the mixture well.

6. Serve immediately.

7. Nutrition Info: Per serving: Calories: 115, Fats: 5.3g, Carbs: 15g, Sugar: 4.6g, Proteins: 5.2g, Sodium: 69mg

Okra Stew with Chicken Andouille Sausage and Shrimp

Servings: 4

Cooking Time: 20 Minutes

Ingredients:

• 3 tablespoons avocado oil, divided

• ½ large onion, halved and then cut into ¼-inch-thick slices

• 8 ounces okra, cut into ½-inch-thick slices

• ¼ teaspoon kosher salt

• ¼ teaspoon freshly ground black pepper

• 3 garlic cloves, minced

• 1 teaspoon dried oregano

• 1 (28-ounce) carton or can chopped tomatoes

• 2 links precooked chicken andouille sausage, cut into ¼-inch-thick slices (about 6 ounces) • 8 ounces raw shrimp (26 to 35 count), peeled and deveined

• Fresh parsley, chopped

Directions:

1. Set the electric pressure cooker to the Sauté setting. When the pot is hot, pour in tablespoons avocado oil.

2. Add the onion and sauté for 3 to 5 minutes or until it

begins to soften.

3. Add the remaining 1½ tablespoons olive oil and okra to the pot. Sprinkle with the salt and pepper. Sauté for 2 to minutes or until the okra begins to brown a little bit. Hit Cancel.

4. Add the garlic, oregano, tomatoes and their juices, and 1 cup of water to the pot. Stir, then close and lock the lid of the pressure cooker. Set the valve to sealing.

5. Cook on high pressure for 20 minutes.

6. When the cooking is complete, hit Cancel and quick release the pressure.

7. Once the pin drops, unlock and remove the lid.

8. Hit Sauté and add the sausage and shrimp to the pot. Cook, uncovered, for about 5 minutes or until the shrimp is opaque and the sausage is hot.

9. Sprinkle with the parsley and serve.

10. Nutrition Info: Per serving(1¼ CUPS): Calories: 252; Total Fat: 12g; Protein: 16g; Carbohydrates: 24g; Sugars: ; Fiber: 6g; Sodium: 732mg

Butter Chicken

Servings: 8

Cooking Time: 25 Minutes

Ingredients:

• 3.5 lbs. chicken drumsticks or thighs

• 1 chopped white onion

• 4 minced garlic cloves

• 2 minced ginger root

• 2 cups water

• 14 oz. full-fat coconut milk

• 6 oz. tomato paste

• 2 tbsps. maple syrup

• ¼ cup cold water

• 4 tbsps. cornstarch

• 1 tbsp. garam masala

• 1 tbsp. curry powder

• 1 tsp. chili powder

• 1¼ tsps. salt

• ½ tsp. black pepper

To Garnish:

• Cilantro

• Green onion

To Serve:

• Brown rice

Directions:

1. Add all the ingredients for the curry starting with the water, onion, garlic, ginger, curry powder, garam masala, chili powder, salt, pepper, coconut milk, tomato paste, maple syrup, and finally the chicken.2. Close and seal the lid, setting the pressure vent to "Sealing" and cook on "Manual, High Pressure" for minutes. It will take the pot about 15 minutes to come to pressure.

3. After 20 minutes, the Pressure Pot will beep, to indicate it is done with the cooking.

4. Allow for a natural pressure release, about 20 minutes, or if you're in a hurry, you can do a quick pressure release by turning the pressure release valve to the "Venting" position, about 2-3 minutes.

5. Carefully open the lid and choose the "Sauté" function.

6. Whisk together the cornstarch and water to form a slurry and pour over the chicken. Stir gently.

7. Cook until the sauce has thickened, and serve with

brown rice, topped with cilantro and green onions.

8. Nutrition Info: Calories 3, Carbs 14g, Fat 17.6 g, Protein 39.2 g, Potassium (K) 725.5 mg, Sodium (Na) 553.2 mg

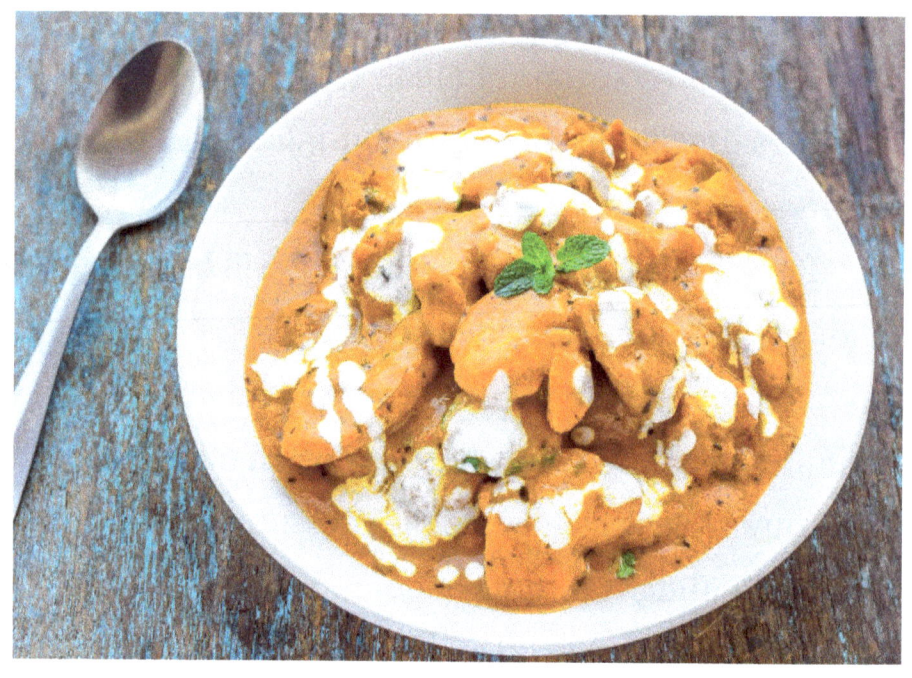

Simple Brown Rice

Servings: 4

Cooking Time: 22 Minutes

Ingredients:

• 1 cup brown basmati rice, rinsed

• 1¼ cups water

• 1 tablespoon olive oil

• Salt, as required

Directions:

1. In the pot of Pressure Pot, place all ingredients and mix well.

2. Close the lid and place the pressure valve to "Seal" position.

3. Press "Manual" and cook under "High Pressure" for about 22 minutes.

4. Press "Cancel" and allow a "Natural" release for about 10 minutes. Then allow a "Quick" release.

5. Open the lid and with a fork, fluff the rice.

6. Serve warm.

7. Nutrition Info: Per serving: Calories: 202, Fats: 4.8g, Carbs: 36.2g, Sugar: 0g, Proteins: 3.6g, Sodium: 41mg

Turkey And Parsnips Curry

Servings: 2

Cooking Time: 20 Minutes

Ingredients:

• 0.5lb parsnip

• 0.5lb chopped cooked turkey

• 1 thinly sliced onion

• 1 cup curry sauce

• 1tbsp oil or ghee

Directions:

1. Set the Pressure Pot to sauté and add the onion and oil.

2. When the onion is soft, add the remaining ingredients and seal.

3. Cook on Stew for 20 minutes.

4. Release the pressure naturally.

5. Nutrition Info: Per serving: Calories: 400; Carbs: 27 ; Sugar: 16 ; Fat: 1; Protein: 43 ; GL: 21

Sweet & Spicy Chicken Breasts

Servings: 4

Cooking Time: 9 Minutes

Ingredients:

- 4 (4-ounce) boneless, skinless chicken breasts
- ¼ cup Yacon syrup
- ½ tablespoon fresh lemon juice
- 1 teaspoon red chili powder
- ½ teaspoon ground coriander
- ½ teaspoon ground cumin
- ½ teaspoon garlic powder
- Ground black pepper, as required
- 1 tablespoon olive oil

Directions:

1. In a large bowl, place all the ingredients except chicken breasts and mix until well combined.
2. Add the chicken breasts and coat with spice mixture generously.
3. Refrigerate for at least minutes.
4. Arrange a steamer trivet in the Pressure Pot and pour 1 cup of water.
5. Place chicken breasts on top of trivet.

6. Close the lid and place the pressure valve to "Seal" position.

7. Press "Manual" and cook under "High Pressure" for about 9 minutes.

8. Press "Cancel" and allow a "Natural" release.

9. Open the lid and serve hot.

10. Nutrition Info: Per serving: Calories: 275, Fats: 12.1g, Carbs: 6.8g, Sugar: 3.7g, Proteins: 33g, Sodium: 112mg

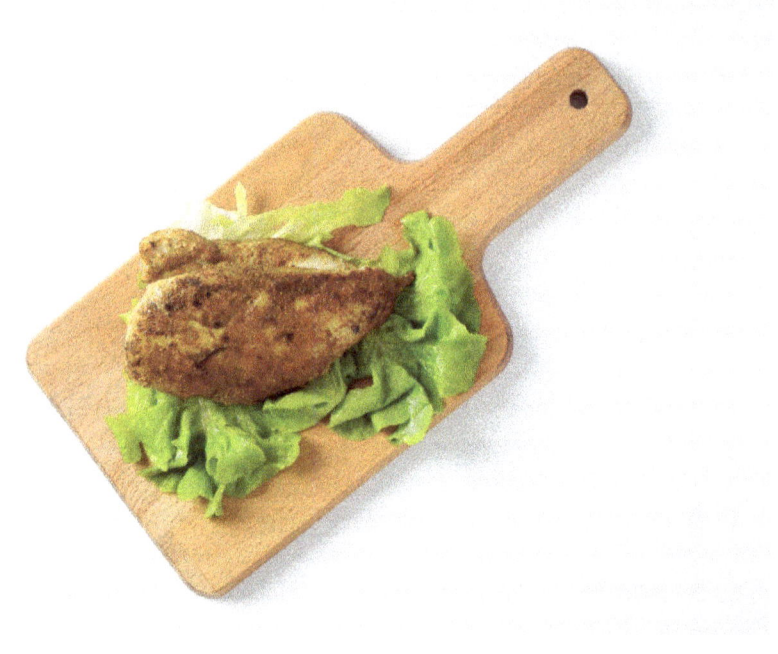

Refried Beans

Servings: 4

Cooking Time: 51 Minutes

Ingredients:

- 1 cup white beans, rinsed and drained
- 1 medium onion, chopped
- 1 jalapeño pepper, minced
- 3 cups water
- 2 garlic cloves, chopped
- 1 bay leaf
- ¼ cup olive oil
- Salt and ground black pepper, as required

Directions:

1. In the pot of Pressure Pot, place the beans, garlic, bay leaf and water and stir to combine.

2. Close the lid and place the pressure valve to "Seal" position.

3. Press "Manual" and cook under "High Pressure" for about 40 minutes.

4. Press "Cancel" and allow a "Natural" release.

5. Open the lid and transfer the beans mixture into a large bowl.

6. With paper towels, pat dry the pot.

7. In the Pressure Pot, place oil and press "Sauté". Now add the onion and jalapeño and cook for about 4-5 minutes.

8. Add the salt and black pepper and cook for about 1-2 minutes.

9. Stir in the bean mixture and with a potato masher, mash the mixture slightly.

10. Cook for about 4 minutes or until the desired thickness of chili.

11. Press "Cancel" and serve hot.

12. Nutrition Info: Per serving: Calories: 182, Fats: 7g, Carbs: 13.8g, Sugar: 1.8g, Proteins: 4.5g, Sodium: 72mg

Pulled Chicken

Servings: 2

Cooking Time: 35 Minutes

Ingredients:

- 1.5lb chicken breast
- 2 shredded onions
- 1 cup low sodium broth
- 1 cup BBQ sauce

Directions:

1. Mix all the ingredients in your Pressure Pot.

2. Cook on Stew for 35 minutes.

3. Release the pressure naturally.

4. Shred the chicken.

5. Nutrition Info: Per serving: Calories: 290; Carbs: 7 ; Sugar: 4 ; Fat: 7 ; Protein: 4; GL: 4

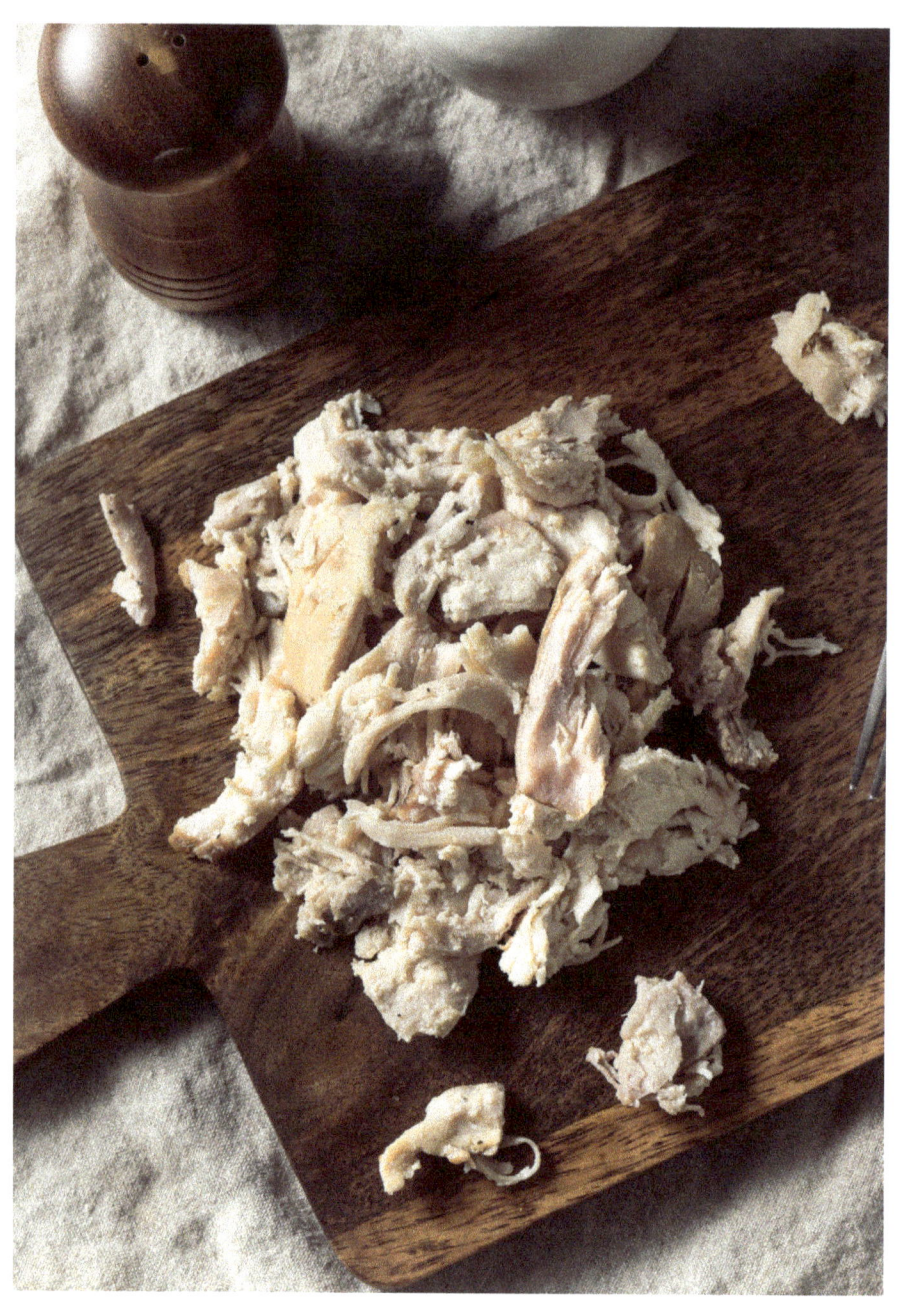

Turkey And Spaghetti Squash

Servings: 2

Cooking Time: 35 Minutes

Ingredients:

- 1lb minced turkey
- 1 cup chicken broth
- 1tbsp mixed Italian herbs
- 1/2 spaghetti squash, to fit the Pressure Pot

Directions:

1. Mix the herbs into the turkey.

2. Pack the turkey into the squash.

3. Pour the broth in your Pressure Pot.

4. Put the squash into the Pressure Pot.

5. Cook on Stew for 3minutes.

6. Release the pressure naturally.

7. Shred the squash and mix the "spaghetti" with the turkey.

8. Nutrition Info: Per serving: Calories: 260; Carbs: 5 ; Sugar: 0 ; Fat: 5 ; Protein: 41 ; GL: 1

Chicken Zoodle Soup

Servings: 2

Cooking Time: 35 Minutes

Ingredients:

• 1lb chopped cooked chicken

• 1lb spiralized zucchini

• 1 cup low sodium chicken soup

• 1 cup diced vegetables

Directions:

1. Mix all the ingredients except the zucchini in your Pressure Pot.

2. Cook on Stew for 35 minutes.

3. Release the pressure naturally.

4. Stir in the zucchini and allow to heat thoroughly.

5. Nutrition Info: Per serving: Calories: 2; Carbs: 5 ; Sugar: 0 ; Fat: 10 ; Protein: 40 ; GL: 1

Chicken With Salsa

Servings: 4

Cooking Time: 20 Minutes

Ingredients:

• 4 (6-ounce) boneless, skinless frozen chicken breasts

• 1 cup homemade tomato puree

• 1 cup mild salsa

• ¼ cup low-fat Parmesan cheese, grated

• 3 tablespoons fresh lime juice

• Ground black pepper, as required

Directions:

1. In the pot of Pressure Pot, place all ingredients except cheese and mix well.

2. Close the lid and place the pressure valve to "Seal" position.

3. Press "Manual" and cook under "High Pressure" for about 12 minutes.

4. Meanwhile, preheat the oven to broiler. Grease a baking dish.

5. Press "Cancel" and carefully allow a "Quick" release.

6. Open the lid and with tongs, transfer the chicken breasts into the prepared baking dish.

7. Now, press "Sauté" of Pressure Pot and cook for about 2-3 minutes or until desired thickness of mixture.

8. Press "Cancel" and pour the sauce over chicken breasts.

9. Sprinkle with cheese and broil for about 4-5 minutes.

10. Serve hot.

11. Nutrition Info: Per serving: Calories: 381, Fats: 14.2g, Carbs: 8.7g, Sugar: 4.8g, Proteins: 52.2g, Sodium: 600mg

Chicken & Beans Chili

Servings: 4

Cooking Time: 13 Minutes

Ingredients:

• 1 pound boneless, skinless chicken breasts

• 30 ounces boiled white northern beans

• 2 jalapeño peppers, hopped

• 1 medium onion, chopped

• 3 cups low-sodium chicken broth

• 2 garlic cloves, minced

• 1 teaspoon dried oregano

• 1 teaspoon ground cumin

• ½ teaspoon red chili powder

• Ground black pepper, as required

Directions:

1. In the pot of Pressure Pot, place all ingredients and mix.

2. Close the lid and place the pressure valve to "Seal" position.

3. Press "Manual" and cook under "High Pressure" for about 1minutes.

4. Press "Cancel" and carefully allow a "Quick" release.

5. Open the lid and with tongs, transfer the chicken thighs into a bowl.

6. With 2 forks, shred the chicken.

7. Return chicken into the pot and stir to combine.

8. Serve immediately.

9. Nutrition Info: Per serving: Calories: 322, Fats: 8.2g, Carbs: 25.1g, Sugar: 1.2g, Proteins: 35g, Sodium: 321mg

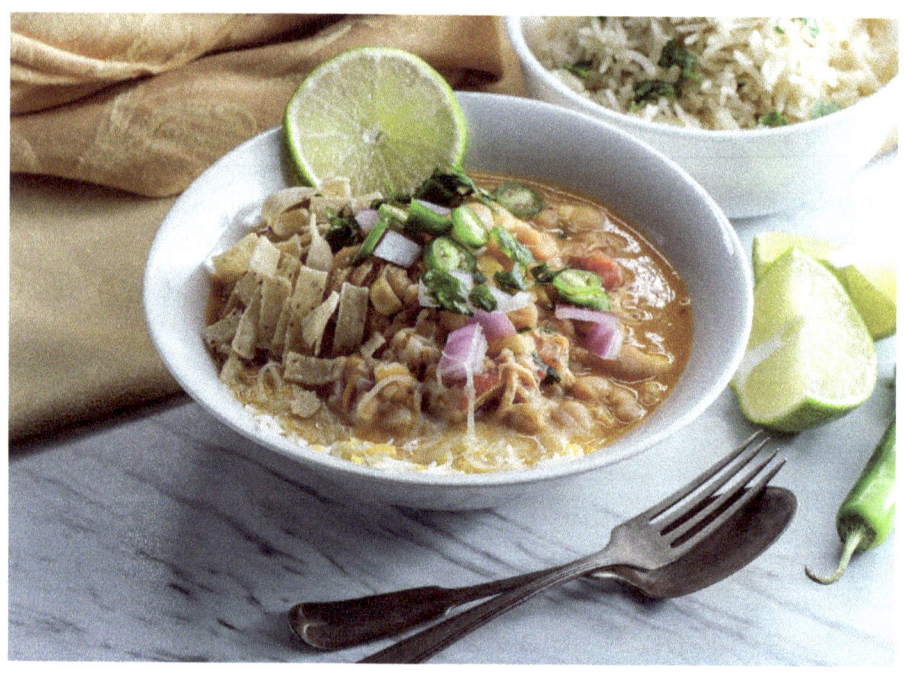

Spinach Stuffed Chicken Breast

Servings: 4

Cooking Time: 20 Minutes

Ingredients:

- 4 chicken breasts
- 4 artichoke heart, chopped
- 4 teaspoons chopped sundried tomato
- 2 teaspoons minced garlic
- ¼ teaspoon ground black pepper
- 1 teaspoon curry powder
- 1 teaspoon paprika
- 20 basil leaves, chopped
- 4-ounce low-fat mozzarella cheese, chopped
- 1 cup water

Directions:

1. Place artichoke heart in a bowl, add tomato, garlic, basil, and mozzarella cheese and stir until mixed.

2. Cut each chicken breast halfway through and then season chicken with salt, black pepper, curry powder, and paprika.

3. Stuff chicken with artichoke mixture and close the filling with chicken using a toothpick.

4. Plugin Pressure Pot, insert the inner pot, pour in water, then insert steamer basket and place stuffed chicken breasts on it.

5. Shut the Pressure Pot with its lid, turn the pressure knob to seal the pot, press the „manual" button, then press the „timer" to set the cooking time to 1minutes and cook at high pressure, Pressure Pot will take 5 minutes or more for building its inner pressure.

6. When the timer beeps, press „cancel" button and do natural pressure release for 10 minutes and then do quick pressure release until pressure nob drops down.

7. Open the Pressure Pot, transfer stuffed chicken to plates and serve.

8. Nutrition Info: Calories: 262 Cal, Carbs: 5 g, Fat: 4.1 g, Protein: 46.1 g, Fiber: 2.4 g.

Chicken Tikka Masala

Servings: 6

Cooking Time: 50 Minutes

Ingredients:

• 2 lbs. diced chicken breasts

• 1 tbsp. unsalted butter

• 1 chopped yellow onion

• 3 minced garlic cloves

• 1 tbsp. minced ginger

• 14 oz. light coconut milk

• 8 oz. no-sodium tomato sauce

• ¾ cup frozen peas

• ½ cup plain non-fat Greek yogurt

• 1 tbsp. garam masala

• 1½ tsp. kosher salt

• 1 tsp. ground chili powder

• 1 tsp. ground turmeric

• 1 tsp. ground cumin

• ¼ tsp. ground cayenne, or to taste

To Serve:

• Chopped cilantro

• Prepared brown rice

Directions:

1. Season the chicken with kosher salt and set it aside.

2. Add butter to the Pressure Pot and select the "Sauté" function.

3. Once the butter has melted, add in the chopped onion, ginger, garlic, ginger, chili powder, garam masala, cayenne, cumin, and turmeric.

4. Sauté until the onion is softened and the spices have bloomed, about 5 minutes.

5. Add the chicken and stir to coat until the outsides of the chicken begin to brown, about 4 minutes.

6. Add the tomato sauce and the reserved ½ a teaspoon of salt. Stir well.

7. Cover and seal the lid, making sure the pressure valve is set to "Sealing."

8. Cook on "Manual, High Pressure" for minutes, and then once cooked, vent to immediately release any remaining pressure.

9. Uncover, stir in the coconut milk, and turn the Pressure Pot back to the "Sauté" function.

10. Simmer for about 15 minutes, until the sauce

slightly thickens.

11. Turn the Pressure Pot off.

12. Site in the peas, cool for 3-4 minutes, and stir in the Greek yogurt.

13. Enjoy warm with naan bread or rice, and a garnish with fresh cilantro.

14. Nutrition Info: Calories 355, Carbs 32g, Fat 10 g, Protein 36 g, Potassium (K) 748 mg, Sodium (Na) 654 mg

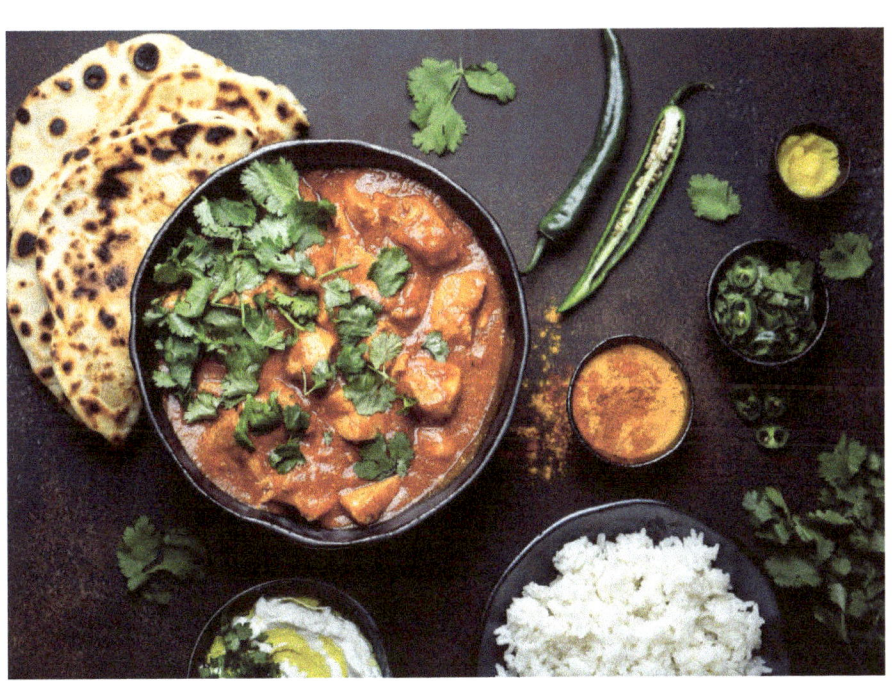

Duck In Orange Sauce

Servings: 2

Cooking Time: 35 Minutes

Ingredients:

• 1lb diced duck breast

• 1lb stir fry vegetables

• 1 cup low sodium broth

• 1 cup orange juice

• 2tbsp marmalade

Directions:

1. Mix all the ingredients in your Pressure Pot.

2. Cook on Stew for 35 minutes.

3. Release the pressure naturally.

4. Nutrition Info: Per serving: Calories: 315; Carbs: 13 ; Sugar: 7 ; Fat: 16 ; Protein: 37 ; GL: 4

Lentils With Lamb

Servings: 10

Cooking Time: 25 Minutes

Ingredients:

- 1-pound lamb, cubed
- 1-pound lentils, dried
- 1-pound red lentils, dried
- 10-ounce frozen spinach
- 14-ounce crushed tomato
- 2 medium white onions, peeled and sliced
- 2 teaspoons minced garlic
- 1 teaspoon grated ginger
- 1 teaspoon salt
- 1 tablespoon ground black pepper
- 1 tablespoon curry powder
- 1 tablespoon ground coriander
- 1 tablespoon ground cumin
- 1 lime, juiced
- 1 cup beef stock
- Water as needed
- 1 cup low-fat yogurt

Directions:

1. Stir together salt, black pepper, curry powder, coriander, and cumin and then sprinkle this spice mix generously on all sides of lamb pieces.

2. Plugin Pressure Pot, insert the inner pot, add seasoned lamb pieces along with remaining ingredients except for yogurt, pour in water to cover all the ingredients and stir until just mixed.

3. Shut the Pressure Pot with its lid, turn the pressure knob to seal the pot, press the „manual" button, then press the „timer" to set the cooking time to 20 minutes and cook at high pressure, Pressure Pot will take 5 minutes or more for building its inner pressure.

4. When the timer beeps, press „cancel" button and do quick pressure release until pressure nob drops down.

5. Open the Pressure Pot, stir lamb and then stir in yogurt.

6. Serve straight away.

7. Nutrition Info: Calories: 126.3 Cal, Carbs: 20.g, Fat: 1.5 g, Protein: 14.6 g, Fiber: 8.9 g.

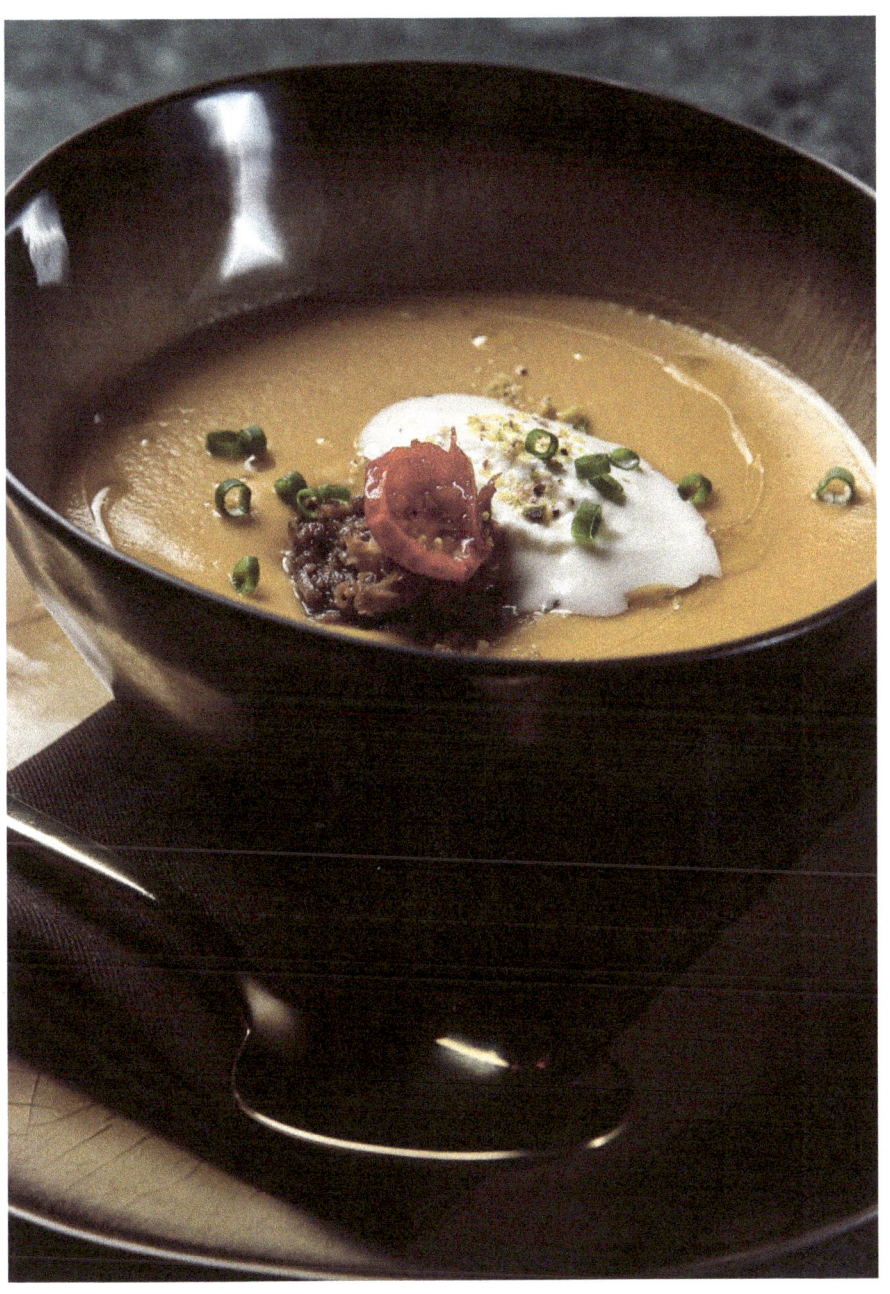

Garlic Herb Chicken

Servings: 4

Cooking Time: 15 Minutes

Ingredients:

- 1-pound chicken breasts
- ½ teaspoon onion powder
- 1 teaspoon garlic powder
- 1 teaspoon salt
- ½ teaspoon ground black pepper
- ½ teaspoon dried thyme
- ½ teaspoon paprika
- ½ teaspoon dried basil
- ¾ cup water

Directions:

1. Stir together salt, black pepper, thyme, paprika, and basil and sprinkle this spice mix generously all over the chicken until evenly coated.

2. Plugin Pressure Pot, insert the inner pot, pour in water, then insert steamer basket and place seasoned chicken on it.

3. Shut the Pressure Pot with its lid, turn the pressure knob to seal the pot, press the „manual" button, then

press the „timer" to set the cooking time to 10 minutes and cook at high pressure, Pressure Pot will take 5 minutes or more for building its inner pressure.

4. When the timer beeps, press „cancel" button and do quick pressure release until pressure nob drops down.

5. Serve straight away.

6. Nutrition Info: Calories: 579 Cal, Carbs: 8 g, Fat: 12 g, Protein: 104 g, Fiber: 1 g.

Turkey Dinner Casserole

Servings: 2

Cooking Time: 10 Minutes

Ingredients:

• 1lb cooked shredded turkey

• 1lb chopped vegetables

• 1 cup low sugar honey mustard sauce

• 1tbsp mixed herbs

• 1 minced onion

Directions:

1. Mix all the ingredients in your Pressure Pot.

2. Cook on Stew for 10 minutes. Release the pressure naturally.

3. Nutrition Info: Per serving: Calories: 400;Carbs: ;Sugar: 18 ;Fat: 13 ;Protein: 39 ;GL: 20

Moroccan Chicken Bowls

Servings: 6

Cooking Time: 25 Minutes

Ingredients:

For the Sweet Potatoes:

- 2 cubed sweet potatoes
- ½ tbsp. olive oil
- 1 tsp. garlic powder
- ½ tbsp. chili powder

For the chicken:

- 3 tbsp. olive oil
- 1½ lbs. chicken thighs
- 1 chopped white onion
- ⅓ cup raisins
- ½ cup chopped green olives
- ½ cup chicken broth
- 1 tbsp. ground cumin
- ½ tbsp. chili powder
- 1 tsp. ginger powder
- 1 tsp. turmeric
- 1½ tsp. garlic powder
- ½ tsp. cayenne

- ⅛ tsp. salt

For the Couscous:

- 1 cup water
- 1 cup couscous
- Zest of 1 lemon
- 2 tbsp. lemon juice
- ¼ cup chopped cilantro
- ¼ cup chopped parsley

To Serve:

- Feta cheese
- Pistachios

Directions:

1. Preheat the oven to 400F.

2. Prepare a baking sheet and then put the sweet potatoes onto the baking sheet.

3. Drizzle the potatoes with olive oil, chili powder, and garlic powder, and mix.

4. Bake for 20-25 minutes.

5. Prepare the marinade for the chicken by mixing the turmeric, cumin, ginger, chili powder, garlic powder, cayenne, and salt.

6. Place the chicken thighs into a bowl and pour over

the spices. Rub, making sure each thigh is well coated, and set aside.

7. Select the "Sauté" function on the Pressure Pot and then add two tablespoons of olive oil.

8. Once hot, place the chicken thighs with the skin side facing down, and cook for 2-3 minutes.

9. Flip over and cook for 2-3 minutes more, before removing from the Pressure Pot.

10. Add all the remaining ingredients for the chicken to the pot, place the chicken on top, and then close and seal your Pressure Pot.

11. Set the Pressure Pot on the "Manual, High Pressure" setting and once the pot is up to pressure, cook for 25 minutes.

12. As the chicken cooks, prepare the couscous.

13. Bring 2 cups of water to a boil.

14. Place the couscous in a bowl and add the boiling water to it.

15. Cover with cling wrap and let rest for 5 minutes. After 5 minutes, uncover the couscous and fluff with a fork.

16. In another large mixing bowl, combine the

ingredients for the couscous, and set them aside.

17. When the chicken is done, the naturally release the pressure, about 5-10 minutes.

18. Carefully uncover and remove the chicken from Pressure Pot and then shred into bits.

19. Discard the skin and bones and return the shredded chicken to the Pressure Pot and mix well with the cooking juices.

20. Serve the chicken with sweet potatoes and couscous, and if desired, top with feta cheese and pistachios.

21. Nutrition Info: Calories 346, Carbs 30g, Fat 15 g, Protein 26 g, Potassium (K) 941.9 mg, Sodium (Na) 239.9 mg

Hoisin Chicken Lettuce Wraps

Servings: 4

Cooking Time: 20 Minutes

Ingredients:

For the chicken

- 2 teaspoons peanut oil
- ⅓ cup low-sodium gluten-free tamari or soy sauce
- 1 tablespoon honey
- 2 tablespoons rice vinegar
- 2 teaspoons Sriracha sauce
- 1 tablespoon minced garlic
- 2 teaspoons peeled and minced fresh ginger
- ⅓ cup Chicken Bone Broth or water
- 2 scallions, both white and green parts, thinly sliced, divided
- 1 bone-in, skin-on chicken breast (about 1 pound)

For the lettuce wraps

- Large lettuce leaves (preferably Bibb)
- 1 cup broccoli slaw or shredded cabbage
- ¼ cup chopped cashews, toasted

Directions:

1. To make the chicken

2. In the electric pressure cooker, whisk together the peanut oil, tamari, honey, rice vinegar, Sriracha, garlic, ginger, and broth. Stir in the white parts of the scallions.

3. Place the chicken breast in the sauce, meat-side down.

4. Close and lock the lid of the pressure cooker. Set the valve to sealing.

5. Cook on high pressure for 20 minutes.

6. When the cooking is complete, hit Cancel and quick release the pressure.

7. Once the pin drops, unlock and remove the lid.

8. Using tongs, transfer the chicken breast to a cutting board. When the chicken is cool enough to handle, remove the skin, shred the chicken, and return it to the pot. Let the chicken soak in the sauce for at least 5 minutes.

9. To make the lettuce wraps

10. Spoon some of the chicken and sauce into the lettuce leaves.

11. Sprinkle with the broccoli slaw, the green parts of the scallions, and the cashews.

12. Serve immediately.

13. Nutrition Info: Per serving: Calories: 233; Total Fat: ; Protein: 14g; Carbohydrates: 18g; Sugars: 10g; Fiber: 2g; Sodium: 1080mg

Duck And Bean Stew

Servings: 2

Cooking Time: 35 Minutes

Ingredients:

• 1lb diced duck breast

• 1lb cooked black beans

• 1 cup low sodium vegetable broth

• 1tbsp 5 spice seasoning

Directions:

1. Mix all the ingredients in your Pressure Pot.

2. Cook on Stew for 35 minutes.

3. Release the pressure naturally.

4. Nutrition Info: Per serving: Calories: 360; Carbs: 16 ; Sugar: 3 ; Fat: 1; Protein: 39 ; GL: 5

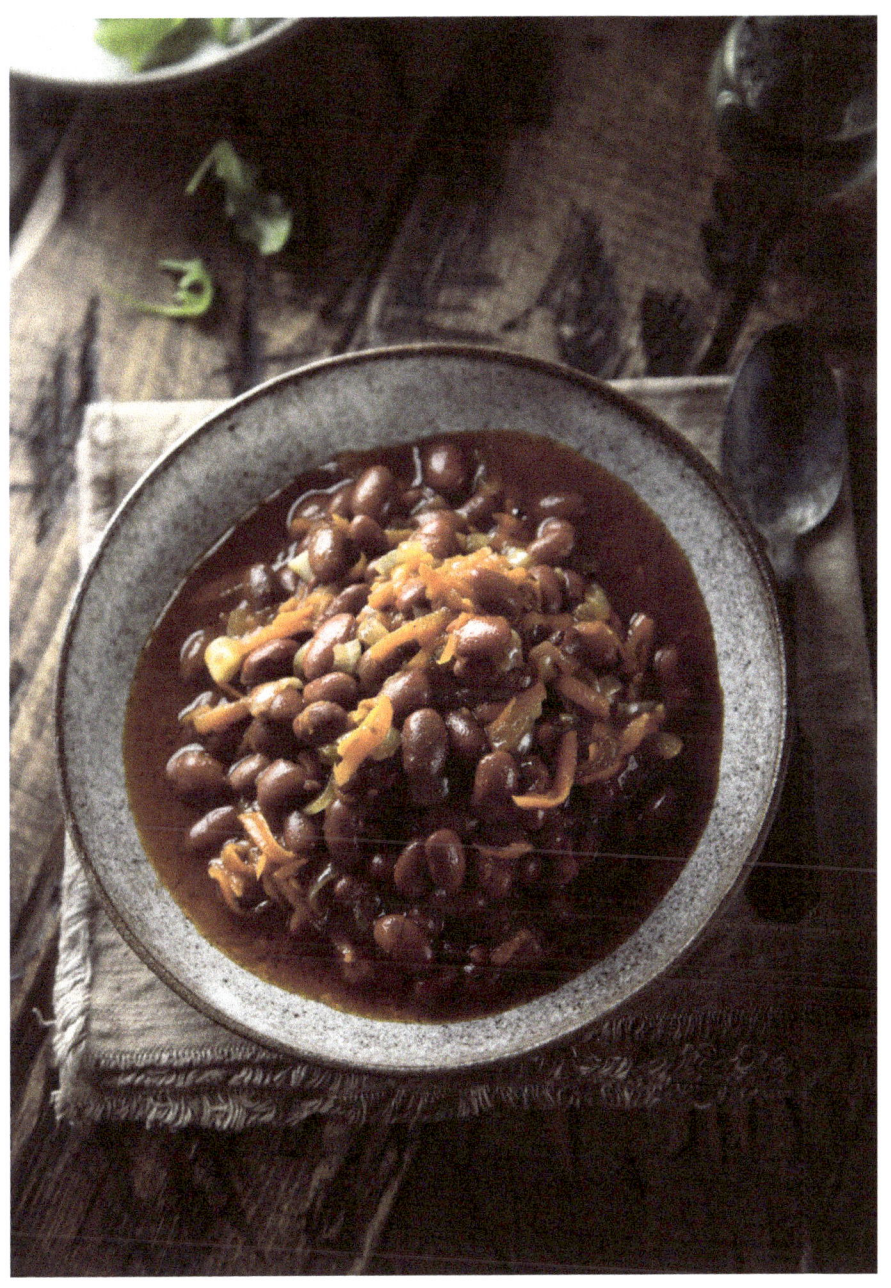

Herbed Whole Turkey Breast

Servings: 12

Cooking Time: 30 Minutes

Ingredients:

• 3 tablespoons extra-virgin olive oil

• 1½ tablespoons herbes de Provence or poultry seasoning

• 2 teaspoons minced garlic

• 1 teaspoon lemon zest (from 1 small lemon)

• 1 tablespoon kosher salt

• 1½ teaspoons freshly ground black pepper

• 1 (6-pound) bone-in, skin-on whole turkey breast, rinsed and patted dry

Directions:

1. In a small bowl, whisk together the olive oil, herbes de Provence, garlic, lemon zest, salt, and pepper.

2. Rub the outside of the turkey and under the skin with the olive oil mixture.

3. Pour 1 cup of water into the electric pressure cooker and insert a wire rack or trivet.

4. Place the turkey on the rack, skin-side up.

5. Close and lock the lid of the pressure cooker. Set the

valve to sealing.

6. Cook on high pressure for 30 minutes.

7. When the cooking is complete, hit Cancel. Allow the pressure to release naturally for 20 minutes, then quick release any remaining pressure.

8. Once the pin drops, unlock and remove the lid.

9. Carefully transfer the turkey to a cutting board. Remove the skin, slice, and serve.

10. Nutrition Info: Per serving: Calories: 146; Total Fat: 9g; Protein: 16g; Carbohydrates: 0g; Sugars: 0g; Fiber: 0g; Sodium: 413mg

Turkey Meatball Stew

Servings: 2

Cooking Time: 35 Minutes

Ingredients:

• 1lb minced turkey

• 1lb chopped vegetables

• 1 cup chicken soup

• 3tbsp almond flour

• 2tbsp mixed seasoning

Directions:

1. Roll the turkey into meatballs with the seasoning and almond flour.

2. Mix all the ingredients in your Pressure Pot.

3. Cook on Stew for minutes.

4. Release the pressure naturally.

5. Nutrition Info: Per serving: Calories: 260; Carbs: 6 ; Sugar: 1 ; Fat: 7 ; Protein: 38 ; GL: 2

Turkey Burger Patty

Servings: 6

Cooking Time: 20 Minutes

Ingredients:

- 2 pounds ground turkey
- 2 teaspoons salt
- 1 teaspoon ground black pepper
- 1 teaspoon red chili powder
- ¾ teaspoon cumin
- 1 cup water

Directions:

1. Place ground turkey in a large bowl, season with salt, black pepper, red chili powder and cumin and then shape mixture into six patties.

2. Plugin Pressure Pot, insert the inner pot, pour in water, and then insert a steamer basket.

3. Wrap each patty with aluminum foil, place them on the steamer basket, then shut the Pressure Pot with its lid and turn the pressure knob to seal the pot.

4. Press the „manual" button, then press the „timer" to set the cooking time to 15 minutes and cook at high pressure, Pressure Pot will take 5 minutes or more for

building its inner pressure.

5. When the timer beeps, press „cancel" button and do quick pressure release until pressure nob drops down.

6. Open the Pressure Pot, remove and uncover patties and serve.

7. Nutrition Info: Calories: 212 Cal, Carbs: 0 g, Fat: 14 g, Protein: 22 g, Fiber: 0 g.

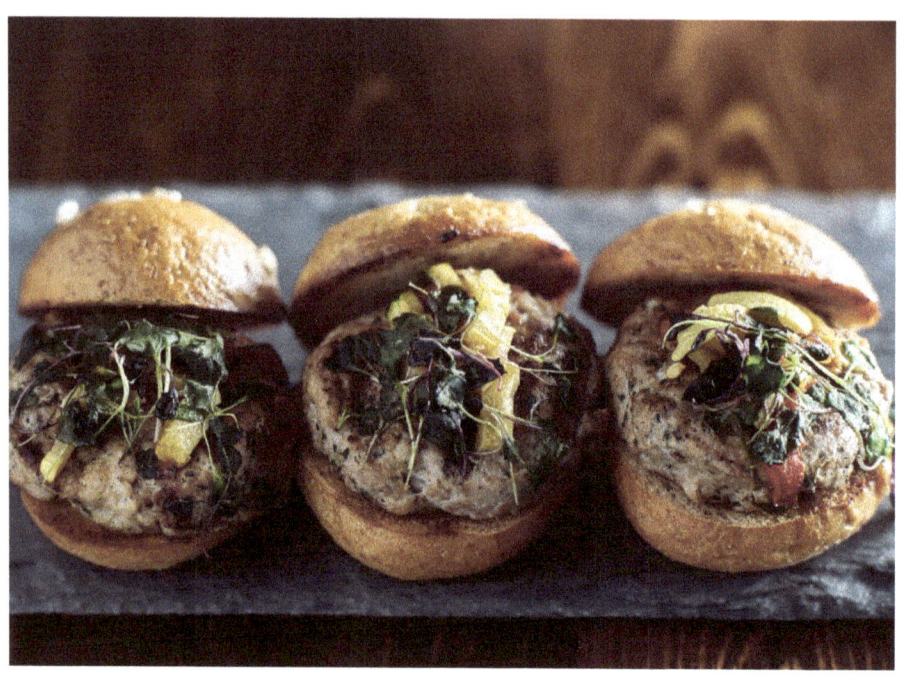

Spicy Cauliflower Rice

Servings: 4

Cooking Time: 14 Minutes

Ingredients:

• 1 medium head cauliflower, chop into large pieces

• 2 tablespoons fresh parsley, chopped

• 2 tablespoons olive oil

• ½ teaspoon dried parsley

• ¼ teaspoon ground cumin

• ¼ teaspoon paprika

• ¼ teaspoon ground turmeric

• Salt, as required

Directions:

1. Arrange a steamer trivet in the Pressure Pot and pour cup of water.

2. Place the cauliflower pieces on top of trivet.

3. Close the lid and place the pressurevalve to "Seal" position.

4. Press "Manual" and cook under "High Pressure" for about 10 minutes.

5. Press "Cancel" and carefully allow a "Quick" release.

6. Open the lid and transfer the cauliflower onto a

plate.

7. Remove the water from Pressure Pot.

8. With paper towels, pat dry the pot.

9. In the Pressure Pot, place oil and press "Sauté". Now add the cooked cauliflower and with a spoon, break into smaller chunks.

10. Add the parsley and spices and cook for about 1-2 minutes.

11.Press "Cancel" and serve hot.

12. Nutrition Info: Per serving: Calories: 79, Fats: 7.2g, Carbs: 3.9g, Sugar: 1.6g, Proteins: 1.4g, Sodium: 60mg

Red Kidney Beans with Spinach

Servings: 4

Cooking Time: 20 Minutes

Ingredients:

- 1 cup red kidney beans, soaked overnight and drained
- 1 cup onion, chopped finely
- ½ cup homemade tomato puree
- 1¼ cups water
- 2 cups fresh spinach, chopped
- 2 tablespoon olive oil
- 1 teaspoon garlic, minced finely
- 1 teaspoon fresh ginger, minced finely
- 1 teaspoon ground coriander
- ½ teaspoon ground turmeric
- 1 teaspoon red chili powder
- Salt, as required

Directions:

1. In the Pressure Pot, place oil and press "Sauté". Now add the onion and cook for about 2 minutes.

2. Add the ginger and garlic and cook for about 30 seconds.

3. Add the tomato puree and spices and cook for about

seconds.

4. Press "Cancel" and stir in the remaining ingredients except spinach.

5. Close the lid and place the pressure valve to "Seal" position.

6. Press "Manual" and cook under and "High Pressure" for about 14 minutes.

7. Press "Cancel" and allow a "Natural" release.

8. Open the lid and press "Sauté".

9. Stir in spinach and lemon juice and cook for about 2-3 mins.

10.Press "Cancel" and serve hot.

11. Nutrition Info: Per serving: Calories: 141, Fats: 7.3g, Carbs: 15.9g, Sugar: 2.9g, Proteins: 5.4g, Sodium: 75mg

Herbed Turkey Breast

Servings: 12

Cooking Time: 55 Minutes

Ingredients:

- 1 (6-pound) boneless, skinless turkey breast
- 1 cup low-sodium chicken broth
- 1 teaspoon dried rosemary, crushed
- 1 teaspoon dried parsley, crushed
- 1 teaspoon dried thyme, crushed
- 1 teaspoon dried sage, crushed
- 1 teaspoon red pepper flakes, crushed
- Ground black pepper, as required

Directions:

1. In a bowl, place the herbs, red pepper flakes and black pepper.

2. Rub turkey breast with herb mixture generously.

3. Arrange a steamer trivet in the Pressure Pot and pour 1½ cups of water.

4. Place the turkey breast on top of trivet.

5. Close the lid and place the pressure valve to "Seal" position.

6. Press "Poultry" and just use the default time of 45

minutes.

7. Press "Cancel" and allow a "Natural" release.

8. Meanwhile, preheat the oven to broiler. Lightly, grease a baking sheet.

9. Open the lid and transfer turkey breast onto prepared baking sheet.

10. Broil for about 5-minutes or until desired doneness of turkey.

11. Remove from oven and place the turkey breast onto a cutting board for about 5-10 minutes.

12. Cut into desired sized slices and serve.

13. Nutrition Info: Per serving: Calories: 263, Fats: 1.1g, Carbs: 0.3g, Sugar: 0g, Proteins: 56.2g, Sodium: 1116mg

Smoky Whole Chicken

Servings: 6

Cooking Time: 26 Minutes

Ingredients:

• 3 ½ pound whole chicken, giblets removed and rinsed

• 1 small onion, cut into four wedges

• 3 teaspoons minced garlic

• 1 tablespoon salt

• 1/4 teaspoon cayenne pepper

• 1 teaspoon ground black pepper

• 1 1/2 teaspoons smoked paprika

• 1/2 teaspoon herbes de Provence

• 2 tablespoons olive oil

• 1 large lemon, halved

• 1 cup Chicken Broth

Directions:

1. Stir together salt, black pepper, cayenne pepper, paprika, herb de Provence and oil and then rub this mixture on the inside and outside of the chicken.

2. Stuff season chicken with onion wedges and lemon halves and tie chicken legs with kitchen twine.

3. Plugin Pressure Pot, insert the inner pot, pour in chicken broth, insert steamer basket and place chicken on it, breast side up.

4. Shut the Pressure Pot with its lid, turn the pressure knob to seal the pot, press the „manual" button, then press the „timer" to set the cooking time to 21 minutes and cook at high pressure, Pressure Pot will take 5 minutes or more for building its inner pressure.

5. When the timer beeps, press „cancel" button and do natural pressure release for 10 minutes and then do quick pressure release until pressure nob drops down.

6. Open the Pressure Pot, transfer chicken to a cutting board and then cut into pieces.

7. Serve straight away.

8. Nutrition Info: Calories: 215 Cal, Carbs: 5 g, Fat: 9 g, Protein: 25 g, Fiber: 1 g.

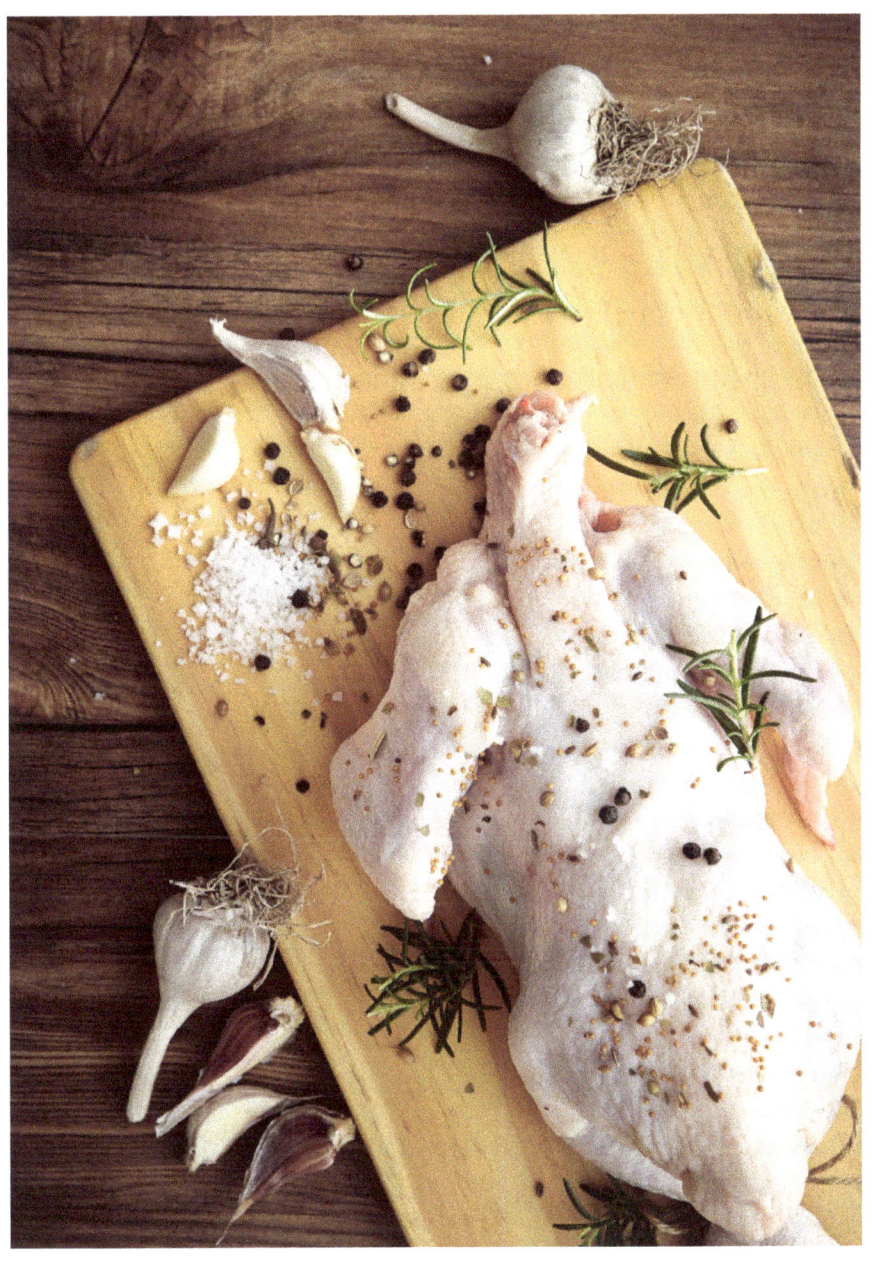

Pesto Chicken and Green Beans

Servings: 4

Cooking Time: 22 Minutes

Ingredients:

- 2 pounds green beans
- 4 medium chicken breasts
- 1 tablespoon garlic salt
- 2 tablespoons lemon pepper seasoning
- 2 tablespoons olive oil
- 6-ounce basil pesto
- 1 ½ cups chicken broth
- 2 cups water

Directions:

1. Place beans in a large bowl, season with lemon pepper, then drizzle with oil and toss until well coated.

2. Plugin Pressure Pot, insert the inner pot, pour in water, then insert steamer basket and place seasoned green beans on it.

3. Shut the Pressure Pot with its lid, turn the pressure knob to seal the pot, press the „manual" button, then press the „timer" to set the cooking time to 2 minutes and cook at low pressure, Pressure Pot will take 5

minutes or more for building its inner pressure.

4. When the timer beeps, press „cancel" button and do quick pressure release until pressure nob drops down.

5. Open the Pressure Pot and divide beans evenly between four plates, set aside until required.

6. Remove steamer basket from the Pressure Pot, rinse the inner pot and pour in chicken broth.

7. Season chicken with garlic salt, add into the Pressure Pot and shut the Pressure Pot with its lid.

8. Turn the pressure knob to seal the pot, press the „poultry" button, then press the „timer" to set the cooking time to 15 minutes and cook at low pressure, Pressure Pot will take 5 minutes or more for building its inner pressure.

9. When the timer beeps, press „cancel" button and do quick pressure release until pressurc nob drops down.

10. Open the Pressure Pot, transfer chicken to a cutting board, let cool for 5 minutes and then shred chicken with two forks.

11. Drizzle pesto over shredded chicken, toss until evenly coated and evenly divide into plates containing green beans.

12. Serve straight away.

13. Nutrition Info: Calories: 415 Cal, Carbs: 14 g, Fat: 16 g, Protein: 49 g, Fiber: 6 g.

Garlicky Broccoli

Servings: 6

Cooking Time: 5 Minutes

Ingredients:

- 1 pound broccoli florets
- 1 jalapeño pepper, chopped finely
- 2 tablespoons olive oil
- 2 garlic cloves, chopped
- ¼ teaspoon red pepper flakes, crushed
- Salt and ground black pepper, as required

Directions:

1. Arrange a trivet in the Pressure Pot and pour cup of water.

2. Place the broccoli florets on top of the trivet in a single layer.

3. Close the lid and place the pressure valve to "Seal" position.

4. Press "Manual" and cook under "High Pressure" for about 3-5 minutes.

5. Press "Cancel" and carefully allow a "Quick" release.

6. Meanwhile, heat the oil in a frying pan over medium heat and sauté the garlic, jalapeño pepper and red

pepper flakes for about 1 minute.

7. Stir in the salt and black pepper and remove from the heat.

8. Open the lid of Pressure Pot and transfer the broccoli onto a serving platter.

9. Drizzle with the garlic mixture and serve immediately.

10. Nutrition Info: Per serving: Calories: , Fats: 7.4g, Carbs: 8.3g, Sugar: 2.1g, Proteins: 3.3g, Sodium: 76mg

Sausage and Cauliflower "grits"

Servings: 4

Cooking Time: 20 Minutes

Ingredients:

• 1 pound frozen (uncooked) Italian-style chicken or turkey sausages • 1 pound frozen riced cauliflower, broken up

• 1 tablespoon extra-virgin olive oil

• Freshly ground black pepper

• ⅓ cup shredded Parmesan cheese

• Chopped fresh parsley, for garnish

Directions:

1. Pour ½ cup of water into the electric pressure cooker and add the sausages.

2. Close and lock the lid of the pressure cooker. Set the valve to sealing.

3. Cook on high pressure for 15 minutes.

4. When the cooking is complete, hit Cancel and quick release the pressure.

5. Once the pin drops, unlock and remove the lid.

6. Using tongs, transfer the sausages to a cutting board and slice into 1-inch rounds. Pour the liquid from the

pot into a measuring cup. Pour ½ cup of the liquid back into the pot; discard the rest.

7. In the electric pressure cooker, combine the sliced sausage, cauliflower, olive oil, and pepper. Close and lock the lid of the pressure cooker. Set the valve to sealing.

8. Cook on high pressure for 5 minutes.

9. When the cooking is complete, hit Cancel and quick release the pressure.

10. Once the pin drops, unlock and remove the lid.

11. Stir in the Parmesan, garnish with parsley, and serve immediately.

12. Nutrition Info: Per serving: Calories: 263; Total Fat: 11g; Protein: 30g; Carbohydrates: 11g; Sugars: 4g; Fiber: 3g; Sodium: 660mg

Mexican Turkey Tenderloin

Servings: 6

Cooking Time: 8 Minutes

Ingredients:

• 1 cup Low-Sodium Salsa or bottled salsa

• 1 teaspoon chili powder

• ½ teaspoon ground cumin

• ¼ teaspoon dried oregano

• 1½ pounds unseasoned turkey tenderloin or boneless turkey breast, cut into 6 pieces • Freshly ground black pepper

• ½ cup shredded Monterey Jack cheese or Mexican cheese blend

Directions:

1. In a small bowl or measuring cup, combine the salsa, chili powder, cumin, and oregano.
Pour half of the mixture into the electric pressure cooker.

2. Nestle the turkey into the sauce. Grind some pepper onto each piece of turkey. Pour the
remaining salsa mixture on top.

3. Close and lock the lid of the pressure cooker. Set the

valve to sealing.

4. Cook on high pressure for 8 minutes.

5. When the cooking is complete, hit Cancel. Allow the pressure to release naturally for 10
 minutes, then quick release any remaining pressure.

6. Once the pin drops, unlock and remove the lid.

7. Sprinkle the cheese on top and put the lid back on for a few minutes to let the cheese melt. 8. Serve immediately.

9. Nutrition Info: Per serving: Calories: 168; Total Fat: 5g; Protein: 28g; Carbohydrates: 3g;
 Sugars: 2g; Fiber: 1g; Sodium: 55g

Chicken Piccata

Servings: 3

Cooking Time: 20 Minutes

Ingredients:

- 1 tbsp. extra-virgin olive oil
- 2 lbs. boneless, skinless chicken breasts
- 1 minced garlic clove
- 4 oz. drained capers
- ¾ cup low-sodium chicken stock
- ¼ cup squeezed lemon juice
- 1 tsp. dried basil
- 1 tsp. dried oregano
- Kosher salt
- Black pepper

Directions:

1. Select the "Sauté" function on your Instant and add oil.

2. Season the chicken and add to the hot Pressure Pot.

3. Brown for about 4 minutes per side and then set aside on a plate.

4. Add the minced garlic and sauté, cooking for about 1 minute, until fragrant.

5. Next, add the lemon juice, broth, basil, and oregano, and deglaze the bottom of the Pressure Pot.

6. Return the seared chicken to Pressure Pot and sprinkle with capers.

7. Cover and seal the Pressure Pot, making sure the pressure valve is set to "Sealing."

8. Cook on the "Manual, High Pressure" setting for 10 minutes.

9. Once done, do a quick pressure release and uncover the pot.

10. Use an instant read meat thermometer; the internal temperature of the chicken should read 165F.

11. Serve immediately with your favorite side.

12. Nutrition Info: Calories 239, Carbs 4g, Fat 8 g, Protein 42 g, Potassium (K) 370 mg, Sodium (Na) 928 mg

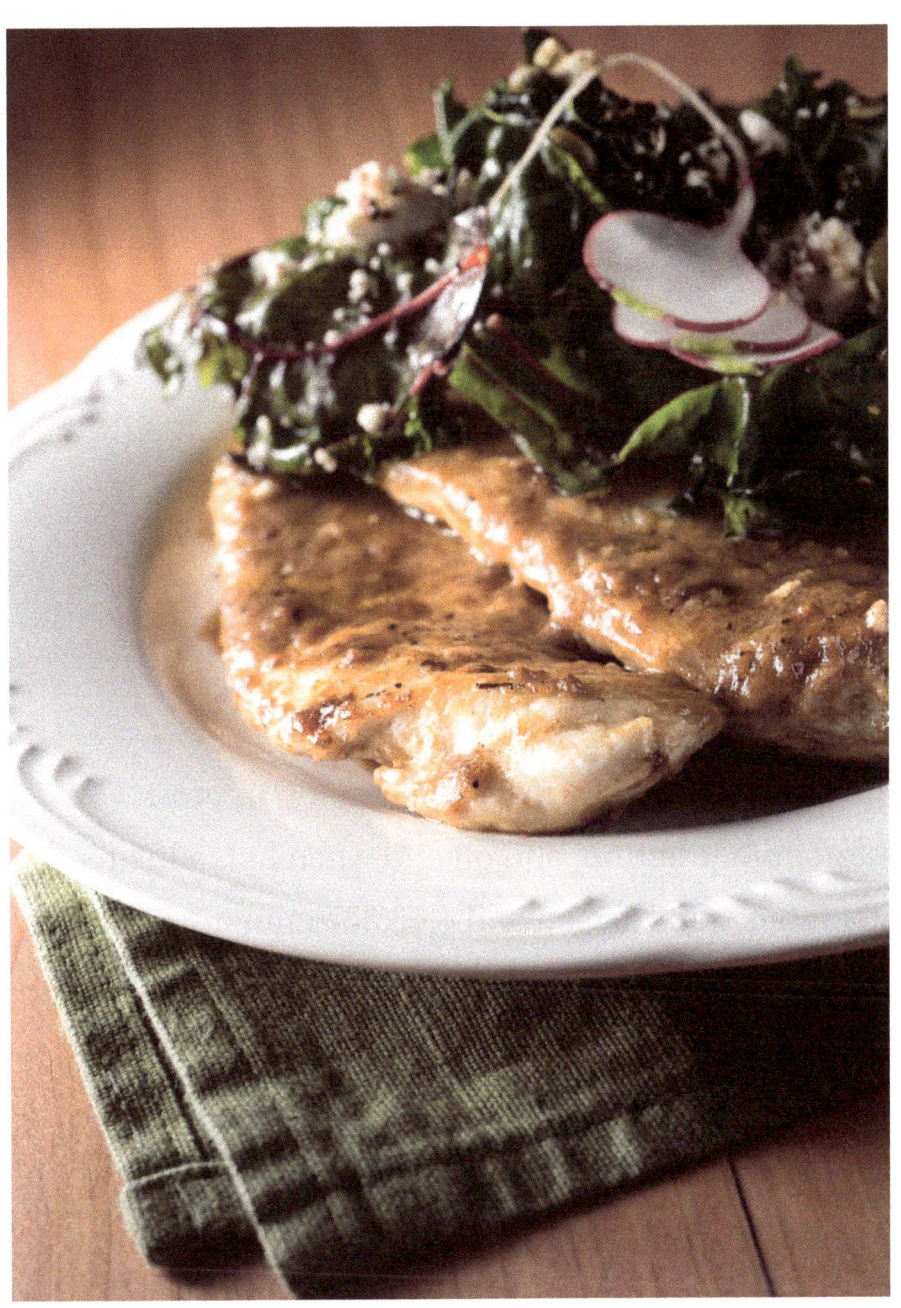

Chicken & Rice

Servings: 6

Cooking Time: 4 Hours And 40 Minutes

Ingredients:

• 1-pound chicken breast

• 3/4 cup brown rice, uncooked

• 1/2-pound mushrooms

• 1/2 cup sliced white onion

• 1/4 teaspoon salt

• 1 tablespoon olive oil

• 1 teaspoon poultry seasoning

• 2 cups chicken broth

Directions:

1. Plugin Pressure Pot, insert the inner pot, press sauté/simmer button, add oil and when hot, add onion, mushroom, and chicken and cook for minutes or more until nicely golden brown on all sides.

2. Add remaining ingredients, except for rice, then press the cancel button, shut the Pressure Pot with its lid and turn the pressure knob to seal the pot.

3. Press the „slow cook" button, then press the „timer" to set the cooking time to 4 hours and cook at low heat

setting.

4. Then transfer chicken to a cutting board, add rice into the Pressure Pot, stir well and continue cooking for 15 minutes or until rice is tender.

5. Meanwhile, let chicken cool for 10 minutes and then shred with two forks.

6. When rice is cooked, return chicken into the Pressure Pot, stir well and continue cooking for 10 minutes or until warm through.

7. Serve straight away.

8. Nutrition Info: Calories: 127 Cal, Carbs: 9.5 g, Fat: 1.2 g, Protein: 19.3 g, Fiber: 0.8 g.

Turkey Zoodles

Servings: 2

Cooking Time: 35 Minutes

Ingredients:

• 1lb diced turkey

• 1lb spiralized zucchini

• 1 cup diced vegetables

• 1 cup low sodium chicken broth

Directions:

1. Mix all the ingredients except the zucchini in your Pressure Pot.

2. Cook on Stew for 35 minutes.

3. Release the pressure naturally.

4. Stir in the zucchini and allow to warm through before serving.

5. Nutrition Info: Per serving: Calories: 2;Carbs: 4 ;Sugar: 0 ;Fat: 7 ;Protein: 39 ;GL: 1

Chickpea Salad

Servings: 6

Cooking Time: 40 Minutes

Ingredients:

- 1 cup chickpeas, dried
- 3 cups water
- 1/4 cup chopped green bell pepper
- 10 black olives, pitted and halved
- 10 cherry tomatoes, halved
- 2 tablespoons chopped cilantro
- 1 medium cucumber, 1/2-inch dice
- 1/2 cup chopped white onion
- 2 tablespoons crumbled feta cheese

For Dressing:

- 1 teaspoon salt
- 1/2 teaspoon ground black pepper
- 1 tablespoon red wine vinegar
- 2 tablespoons olive oil

Directions:

1. Plugin Pressure Pot, insert the inner pot, add chickpeas, and pour in water.

2. Shut the Pressure Pot with its lid, turn the pressure

knob to seal the pot, press the „manual" button, then press the „timer" to set the cooking time to 35 minutes and cook at high pressure, Pressure Pot will take 5 minutes or more for building its inner pressure.

3. Meanwhile, whisk together all the ingredients for the dressing and set aside until required.

4. When the timer beeps, press „cancel" button and do quick pressure release until pressure nob drops down.

5. Open the Pressure Pot, drain the chickpeas, let cool for 20 minutes and then transfer into a salad bowl.

6. Drizzle chickpeas with prepared salad dressing, then add remaining ingredients and toss until well coated.

7. Chill salad in the refrigerator for 30 minutes and then serve.

8. Nutrition Info: Calories: 301 Cal, Carbs: 37 g, Fat: 13 g, Protein: 11 g, Fiber: 10 g.

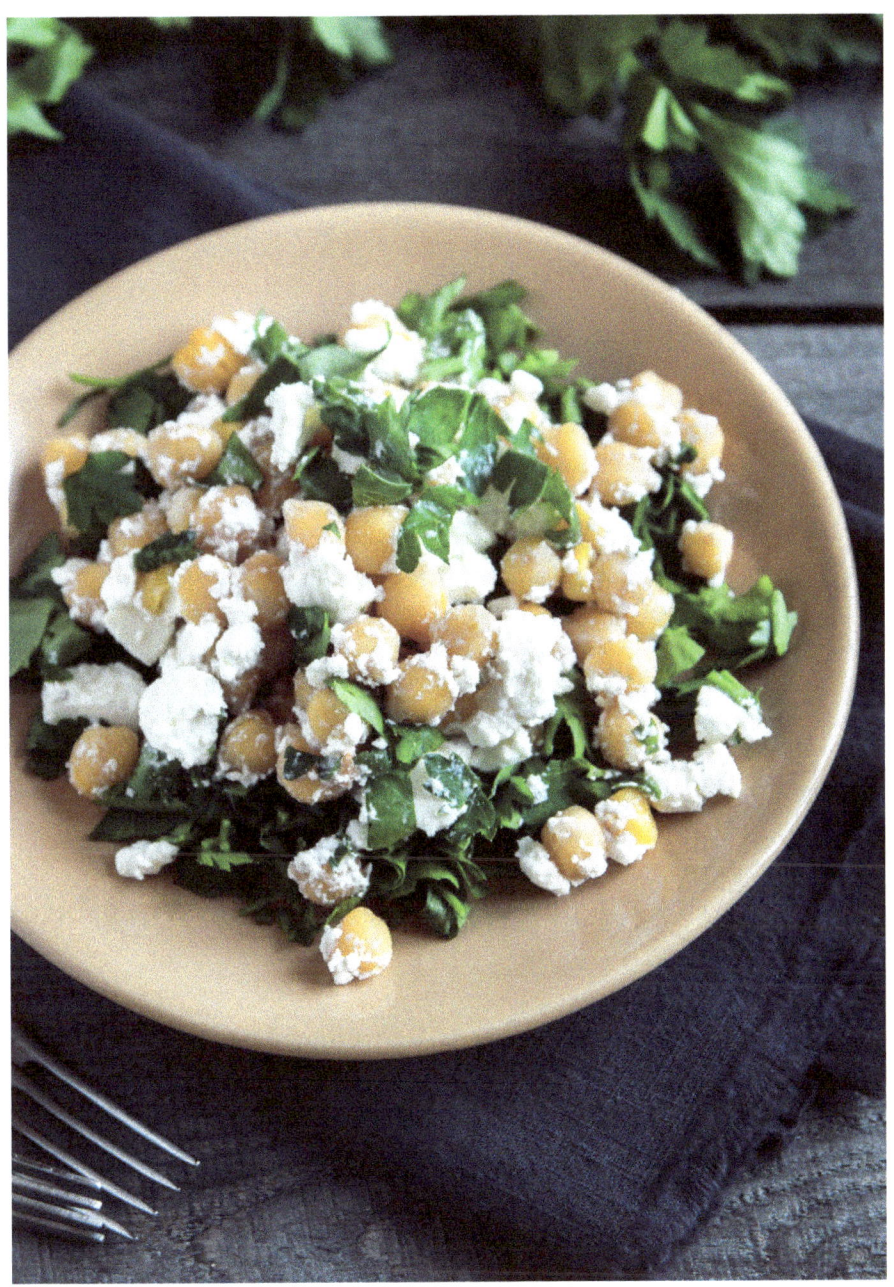

Coffee-steamed Carrots

Servings: 4

Cooking Time: 3 Minutes

Ingredients:

• 1 cup brewed coffee

• 1 teaspoon light brown sugar

• ½ teaspoon kosher salt

• Freshly ground black pepper

• 1 pound baby carrots

• Chopped fresh parsley

• 1 teaspoon grated lemon zest

Directions:

1. Pour the coffee into the electric pressure cooker. Stir in the brown sugar, salt, and pepper.
Add the carrots.

2. Close and lock the lid of the pressure cooker. Set the valve to sealing.

3. Cook on high pressure for minutes.

4. When the cooking is complete, hit Cancel and quick release the pressure.

5. Once the pin drops, unlock and remove the lid.

6. Using a slotted spoon, transfer the carrots to a

serving bowl. Sprinkle with the parsley and lemon zest and serve.

7. Nutrition Info: Per serving: Calories: 51; Total Fat: 0g; Protein: 1g; Carbohydrates: 12g; Sugars: ; Fiber: 4g; Sodium: 344mg

Rosemary Potatoes

Servings: 2

Cooking Time: 25 Minutes.

Ingredients:

• 1lb red potatoes

• 1 cup vegetable stock

• 2tbsp olive oil

• 2tbsp rosemary sprigs

Directions:

1. Put the potatoes in the steamer basket and add the stock into the Pressure Pot.

2. Steam the potatoes in your Pressure Pot for 15 minutes.

3. Depressurize and pour away the remaining stock.

4. Set to sauté and add the oil, rosemary, and potatoes.

5. Cook until brown.

6. Nutrition Info: Per serving: Calories: 195;Carbs: 31 ;Sugar: 1 ;Fat: ;Protein: 5 ;GL: 25

Corn on the Cob

Servings: 12

Cooking Time: 5 Minutes

Ingredients:

• 6 ears corn

Directions:

1. Remove the husks and silk from the corn. Cut or break each ear in half.

2. Pour 1 cup of water into the bottom of the electric pressure cooker. Insert a wire rack or trivet.

3. Place the corn upright on the rack, cut side down. Close and lock the lid of the pressure cooker. Set the valve to sealing.

4. Cook on high pressure for 5 minutes.

5. When the cooking is complete, hit Cancel and quick release the pressure.

6. Once the pin drops, unlock and remove the lid.

7. Use tongs to remove the corn from the pot. Season as desired and serve immediately.

8. Nutrition Info: Per serving(½ EAR OF CORN): Calories: 62; Total Fat: 1g; Protein: 2g; Carbohydrates: 14g; Sugars: 5g; Fiber: 1g; Sodium: 11mg

Chili Lime Salmon

Servings: 2

Cooking Time: 10 Minutes

Ingredients:

For Sauce:

- 1 jalapeno pepper, deseeded and diced
- 1 tablespoon chopped parsley
- 1 teaspoon minced garlic
- 1/2 teaspoon cumin
- 1/2 teaspoon paprika
- 1/2 teaspoon lime zest
- 1 tablespoon honey
- 1 tablespoon lime juice
- 1 tablespoon olive oil
- 1 tablespoon water

For Fish:

- 2 salmon fillets, each about 5 ounces
- 1 cup water
- 1/2 teaspoon salt
- 1/8 teaspoon ground black pepper

Directions:

1. Prepare salmon and for this, season salmon with salt

and black pepper until evenly coated.

2. Plugin Pressure Pot, insert the inner pot, pour in water, then place steamer basket and place seasoned salmon on it.

3. Shut the Pressure Pot with its lid, turn the pressure knob to seal the pot, press the „steam" button, then press the „timer" to set the cooking time to 5 minutes and cook at high pressure, Pressure Pot will take 5 minutes or more for building its inner pressure.

4. Meanwhile, place all the ingredients for the sauce in a bowl, whisk until combined and set aside until required.

5. When the timer beeps, press „cancel" button and do quick pressure release until pressure nob drops down.

6. Open the Pressure Pot, then transfer salmon to a serving plate and drizzle generously with prepared sauce.7. Serve straight away.

 8. Nutrition Info: Calories: 305 Cal, Carbs: 29 g, Fat: 5 g, Protein: 36 g, Fiber: g.

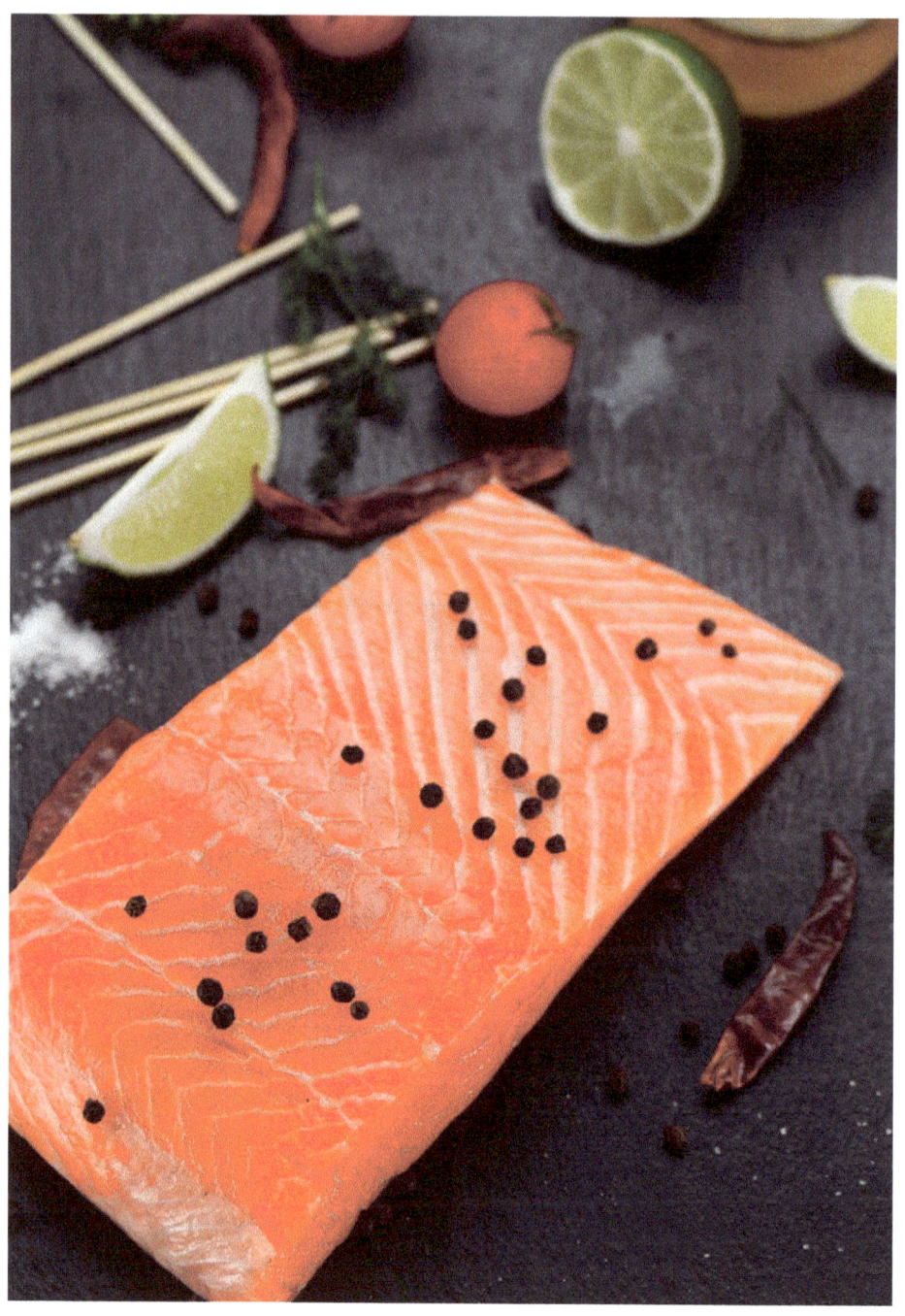

Collard Greens

Servings: 12

Cooking Time: 6 Hours And 5 Minutes

Ingredients:

- 2 pounds chopped collard greens
- ¾ cup chopped white onion
- 1 teaspoon onion powder
- 1 teaspoon garlic powder
- 1 teaspoon salt
- 2 teaspoons brown sugar
- ½ teaspoon ground black pepper
- ½ teaspoon red chili powder
- ¼ teaspoon crushed red pepper flakes
- 3 tablespoons apple cider vinegar
- 2 tablespoons olive oil
- 14.5-ounce vegetable broth
- 1/2 cup water

Directions:

1. Plugin Pressure Pot, insert the inner pot, add onion and collard, then pour in vegetable broth and water.

2. Shut the Pressure Pot with its lid, turn the pressure knob to seal the pot, press the „slow cook" button, then

press the „timer" to set the cooking time to 6 hours at high heat setting.

3. When the timer beeps, press „cancel" button and do natural pressure release until pressure nob drops down.

4. Open the Pressure Pot, add remaining ingredients and stir until mixed.

5. Then press the „sauté/simmer" button and cook for 3 to minutes or more until collards reach to desired texture.

6. Serve straight away.

7. Nutrition Info: Calories: 49.6 Cal, Carbs: 2.3 g, Fat: 3.1 g, Protein: 3.4 g, Fiber: 0.5 g.

Creamy Sweet Potato Soup

Servings: 6

Cooking Time: 10 Minutes

Ingredients:

- 2 tablespoons avocado oil
- 1 small onion, chopped
- 2 celery stalks, chopped
- 2 teaspoons minced garlic
- 1 teaspoon kosher salt
- ½ teaspoon freshly ground black pepper
- 1 teaspoon ground turmeric
- ½ teaspoon ground cinnamon
- 2 pounds sweet potatoes, peeled and cut into 1-inch cubes
- 3 cups Vegetable Broth or Chicken Bone Broth
- Plain Greek yogurt, to garnish (optional)
- Chopped fresh parsley, to garnish (optional)
- Pumpkin seeds (pepitas), to garnish (optional)

Directions:

1. Set the electric pressure cooker to the Sauté setting. When the pot is hot, pour in the avocado oil.

2. Sauté the onion and celery for 3 to 5 minutes or until

the vegetables begin to soften.

3. Stir in the garlic, salt, pepper, turmeric, and cinnamon. Hit Cancel.

4. Stir in the sweet potatoes and broth.

5. Close and lock the lid of the pressure cooker. Set the valve to sealing.

6. Cook on high pressure for 10 minutes.

7. When the cooking is complete, hit Cancel and allow the pressure to release naturally.

8. Once the pin drops, unlock and remove the lid.

9. Use an immersion blender to purée the soup right in the pot. If you don't have an immersion blender, transfer the soup to a blender or food processor and purée. (Follow the instructions that came with your machine for blending hot foods.)

10. Spoon into bowls and serve topped with Greek yogurt, parsley, and/or pumpkin seeds (if using).

11. Nutrition Info: Per serving(1 CUP): Calories: 193; Total Fat: 5g; Protein: 3g; Carbohydrates: 36g; Sugars: 8g; Fiber: 6g; Sodium: 302mg

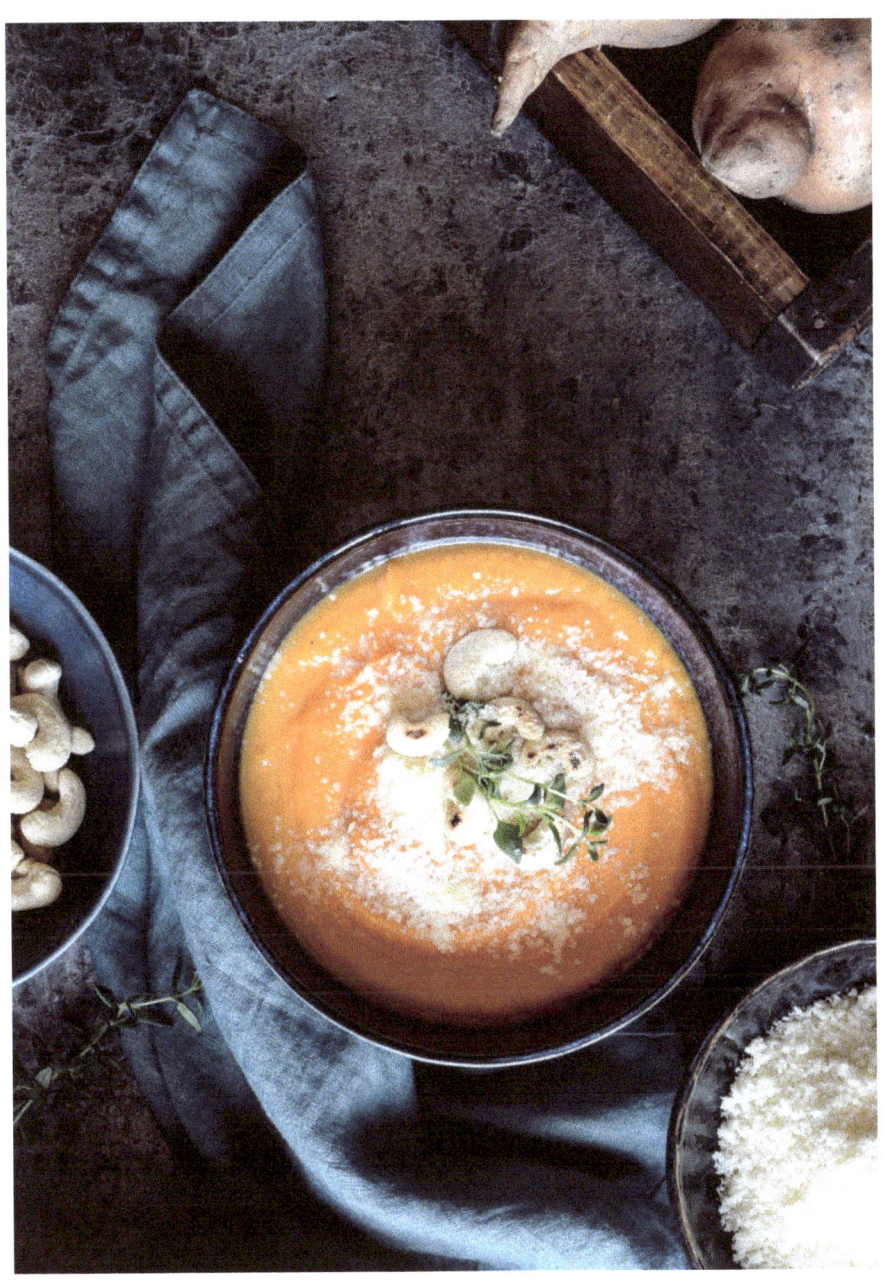

Mashed Pumpkin

Servings: 2

Cooking Time: 15 Minutes

Ingredients:

• 2 cups chopped pumpkin

• 0.5 cup water

• 2tbsp powdered sugar-free sweetener of choice

• 1tbsp cinnamon

Directions:

1. Place the pumpkin and water in your Pressure Pot.

2. Seal and cook on Stew 15 minutes.

3. Remove and mash with the sweetener and cinnamon.

4. Nutrition Info: Per serving: Calories: 12;Carbs: 3 ;Sugar: 1 ;Fat: 0 ;Protein: 0 ;GL: 1

Chicken Noodle Soup

Servings: 12

Cooking Time: 20 Minutes

Ingredients:

• 2 tablespoons avocado oil

• 1 medium onion, chopped

• 3 celery stalks, chopped

• 1 teaspoon kosher salt

• ¼ teaspoon freshly ground black pepper

• 2 teaspoons minced garlic

• 5 large carrots, peeled and cut into ¼-inch-thick rounds

• 3 pounds bone-in chicken breasts (about 3)

• 4 cups Chicken Bone Broth or low-sodium store-bought chicken broth

• 4 cups watcr

• 2 tablespoons soy sauce

• 6 ounces whole grain wide egg noodles

Directions:

1. Set the electric pressure cooker to the Sauté setting. When the pot is hot, pour in the avocado oil.

2. Sauté the onion, celery, salt, and pepper for 3 to 5

minutes or until the vegetables begin to soften.

3. Add the garlic and carrots and stir to mix well. Hit Cancel.

4. Add the chicken to the pot, meat-side down. Add the broth, water, and soy sauce. Close and lock the lid of the pressure cooker. Set the valve to sealing.

5. Cook on high pressure for 20 minutes.

6. When the cooking is complete, hit Cancel and quick release the pressure. Unlock and remove the lid.

7. Using tongs, remove the chicken breasts to a cutting board. Hit Sauté/More and bring the soup to a boil.

8. Add the noodles and cook for 4 to 5 minutes or until the noodles are al dente.

9. While the noodles are cooking, use two forks to shred the chicken. Add the meat back to the pot and save the bones to make more bone broth.

10. Season with additional pepper, if desired, and serve.

11. Nutrition Info: Per serving(1 CUP): Calories: 330; Total Fat: 15g; Protein: 32g; Carbohydrates: 17g; Sugars: 3g; Fiber: 4g; Sodium: 451mg

Buttercup Squash Soup

Servings: 6

Cooking Time: 10 Minutes

Ingredients:

- 2 tablespoons extra-virgin olive oil
- 1 medium onion, chopped
- 4 to 5 cups Vegetable Broth or Chicken Bone Broth
- 1½ pounds buttercup squash, peeled, seeded, and cut into 1-inch chunks
- ½ teaspoon kosher salt
- ¼ teaspoon ground white pepper
- Whole nutmeg, for grating

Directions:

1. Set the electric pressure cooker to the Sauté setting. When the pot is hot, pour in the olive oil.

2. Add the onion and sauté for 3 to 5 minutes, until it begins to soften. Hit Cancel.

3. Add the broth, squash, salt, and pepper to the pot and stir. (If you want a thicker soup, use 4 cups of broth. If you want a thinner, drinkable soup, use 5 cups.)

4. Close and lock the lid of the pressure cooker. Set the

valve to sealing.

5. Cook on high pressure for 10 minutes.

6. When the cooking is complete, hit Cancel and allow the pressure to release naturally.

7. Once the pin drops, unlock and remove the lid.

8. Use an immersion blender to purée the soup right in the pot. If you don't have an immersion blender, transfer the soup to a blender or food processor and purée. (Follow the instructions that came with your machine for blending hot foods.)

9. Pour the soup into serving bowls and grate nutmeg on top.

10.Nutrition Info: Per serving(1⅓ CUPS): Calories: 1 Total Fat: 5g; Protein: 1g; Carbohydrates: 18g; Sugars: 4g; Fiber: 4g; Sodium: 166mg.

Tuna Melt

Servings: 2

Cooking Time: 10 Minutes

Ingredients:

- 8-ounce tuna fillet
- 2 whole-wheat English muffins, halved
- 1 green onion, sliced
- ½ teaspoon ground black pepper
- 1 tablespoon dried dill weed
- 1 tablespoon Dijon mustard
- 3/4 cup Coleslaw mix
- 1 ½ tablespoons mayonnaise
- 1/3 cup grated cheddar cheese
- 1 cup water

Directions:

1. Plugin Pressure Pot, insert the inner pot, pour in water, then insert steamer basket and place tuna on it.

2. Shut the Pressure Pot with its lid, turn the pressure knob to seal the pot, press the „steam" button, then press the „timer" to set the cooking time to 4 minutes and cook at high pressure, Pressure Pot will take 5 minutes or more for building its inner pressure.

3. Meanwhile, place remaining ingredients except for cheese and muffins in a large bowl and stir until mixed.

4. When the timer beeps, press „cancel" button and do natural pressure release for 5 minutes and then do quick pressure release until pressure nob drops down.

5. Open the Pressure Pot, then transfer tuna to a cutting board, let cool for 10 minutes and then shred with two forks.

6. Add shredded tuna to mayonnaise mixture and stir until combined.

7. Cut muffins into half, then top evenly with tuna mixture and sprinkle with cheese.

8. Place muffins under the broiler and cook for 4 to 5 minutes or until cheese melts.

9. Serve straight away.

10. Nutrition Info: Calories: 306.1 Cal, Carbs: 27.5 g, Fat: 5.5 g, Protein: 35 g, Fiber: 3.8 g.

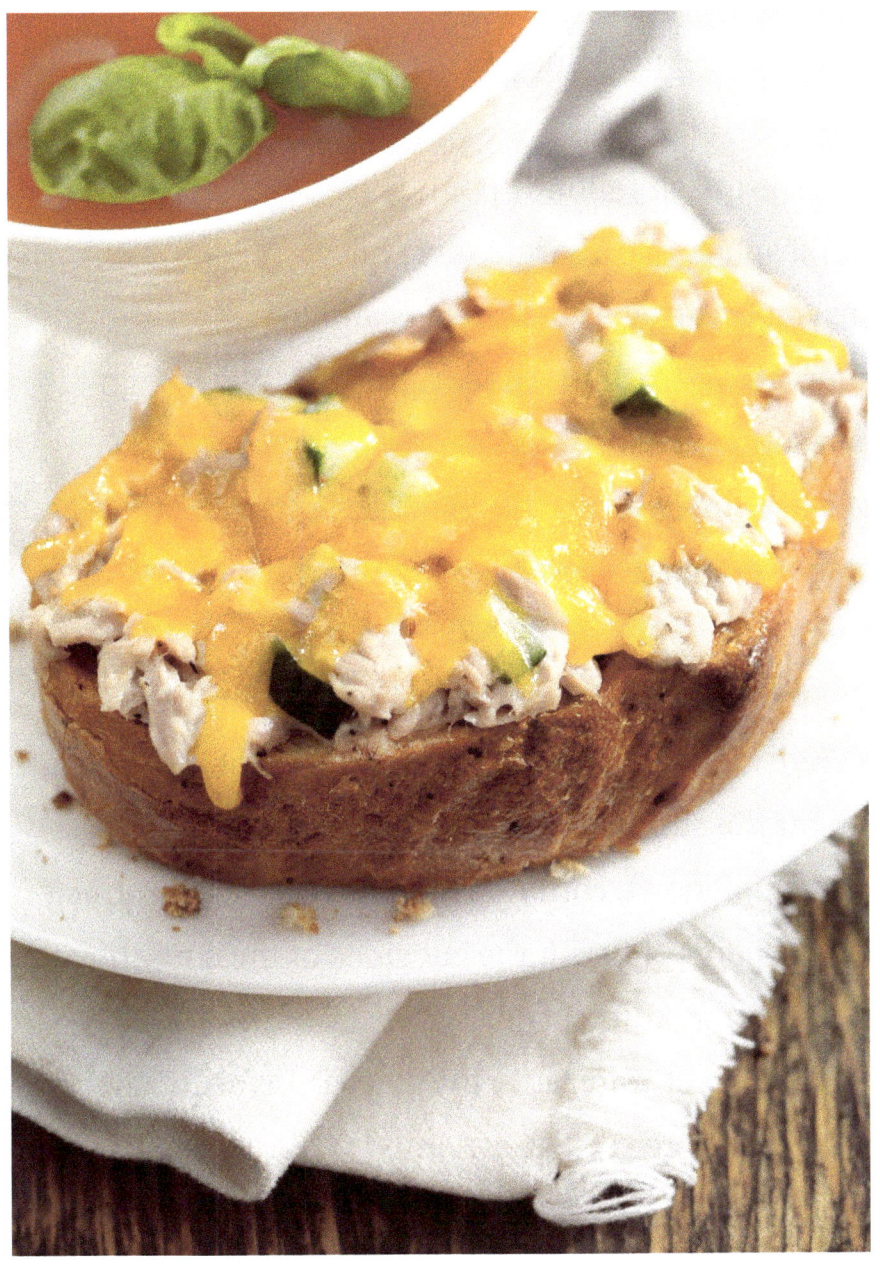

Parmesan-topped Acorn Squash

Servings: 4

Cooking Time: 20 Minutes

Ingredients:

- 1 acorn squash (about 1 pound)
- 1 tablespoon extra-virgin olive oil
- 1 teaspoon dried sage leaves, crumbled
- ¼ teaspoon freshly grated nutmeg
- ⅛ teaspoon kosher salt
- ⅛ teaspoon freshly ground black pepper
- 2 tablespoons freshly grated Parmesan cheese

Directions:

1. Cut the acorn squash in half lengthwise and remove the seeds. Cut each half in half for a total of 4 wedges. Snap off the stem if it's easy to do.

2. In a small bowl, combine the olive oil, sage, nutmeg, salt, and pepper. Brush the cut sides of the squash with the olive oil mixture.

3. Pour 1 cup of water into the electric pressure cooker and insert a wire rack or trivet.

4. Place the squash on the trivet in a single layer, skin-side down.

5. Close and lock the lid of the pressure cooker. Set the valve to sealing.

6. Cook on high pressure for 20 minutes.

7. When the cooking is complete, hit Cancel and quick release the pressure.

8. Once the pin drops, unlock and remove the lid.

9. Carefully remove the squash from the pot, sprinkle with the Parmesan, and serve.

10. Nutrition Info: Per serving: Calories: 85; Total Fat: 4g; Protein: 2g; Carbohydrates: 12g; Sugars: 0g; Fiber: 2g; Sodium: 282mg

Quinoa Tabbouleh

Servings: 6

Cooking Time: 16 Minutes

Ingredients:

- 1 cup quinoa, rinsed
- 1 large English cucumber, cut into ¼-inch pieces
- 2 scallions, sliced
- 2 cups cherry tomatoes, halved
- 2/3 cup chopped parsley
- 1/2 cup chopped mint
- ½ teaspoon minced garlic
- 1/2 teaspoon salt
- ½ teaspoon ground black pepper
- 2 tablespoon lemon juice
- 1/2 cup olive oil

Directions:

1. Plugin Pressure Pot, insert the inner pot, add quinoa, then pour in water and stir until mixed.

2. Shut the Pressure Pot with its lid and turn the pressure knob to seal the pot.

3. Press the "manual" button, then press the „timer" to set the cooking time to 1 minute and cook at high

pressure, Pressure Pot will take 5 minutes or more for building its inner pressure.

4. When the timer beeps, press „cancel" button and do natural pressure release for 10 minutes and then do quick pressure release until pressure nob drops down.

5. Open the Pressure Pot, fluff quinoa with a fork, then spoon it on a rimmed baking sheet, spread quinoa evenly and let cool.

6. Meanwhile, place lime juice in a small bowl, add garlic and stir until just mixed.

7. Then add salt, black pepper, and olive oil and whisk until combined.

8. Transfer cooled quinoa to a large bowl, add remaining ingredients, then drizzle generously with the prepared lime juice mixture and toss until evenly coated.

9. Taste quinoa to adjust seasoning and then serve.

 10. Nutrition Info: Calories: 283.6 Cal, Carbs: 30.6 g, Fat: 16.1 g, Protein: 5.8 g, Fiber: 3.4 g.

Lightning Source UK Ltd.
Milton Keynes UK
UKHW021443200721
387459UK00004B/38